NATURAL THERAPY FOR YOUR LIVER

CHRISTOPHER HOBBS

NATURAL THERAPY FOR YOUR LIVER

SECOND EDITION

Herbs and Other Natural Remedies

for a Healthy Liver

AVERY

a member of Penguin Putnam Inc.

New York

Most Avery books are available at special quantity discounts for bulk purchase for sales promotions, premiums, fund-raising, and educational needs. Special books or book excerpts also can be created to fit specific needs. For details, write Putnam Special Markets, 375 Hudson Street, New York, NY 10014.

a member of
Penguin Putnam Inc.
375 Hudson Street
New York, NY 10014
www.penguinputnam.com

Copyright © 1986, 2002 by Christopher Hobbs
Plant illustrations by Donna Cehrs
Anatomy illustration by Prancine Martin

Library of Congress Cataloging-in-Publication Data

Hobbs, Christopher, date.
Natural therapy for your liver : herbs and other natural
remedies for a healthy liver / Christopher Hobbs.
p.   cm.
Includes index.
ISBN 1-58333-132-8
1. Liver—Diseases—Alternative treatment.   2. Naturopathy.
3. Alternative medicine.   I. Title.
RC846 .H635   2002   2002018262
616.3'6206—dc21

Printed in the United States of America
13   15   17   19   20   18   16   14

BOOK DESIGN BY RENATO STANISIC

CONTENTS

INTRODUCTION TO THE
SECOND EDITION

A remarkable organ, the liver is largely unappreciated for the more than one hundred separate body functions it performs. It has been said that it is not called the live-r for nothing: It keeps us living. Keeping the liver healthy and functioning smoothly is considered a basic principle of natural medicine by both doctors and herbalists. A major organ of digestion and assimilation, the liver processes the nutrients the body needs to maintain health and repair diseased or damaged tissue, and eliminates toxic wastes from the body.

Unfortunately, liver disease is currently the third most common cause of death for people between the ages of twenty-five and fifty-nine, and is the seventh overall. Each year, more than 27,000 people in the United States die of cirrhosis of the liver, a tragic situation that could be prevented with a proper diet and natural liver therapy.

The aim of this book is to present practical, up-to-date information about effective ways to regain and maintain optimal liver health. Specifically, we will look at:

- The functions of the liver as defined by Western science as well as by Traditional Chinese Medicine
- The ways in which fat, oils, and other common foods affect the liver
- An optimum diet for maintaining the highest liver health and specific dietary recommendations for common liver ailments
- Herbal remedies for a variety of liver disorders
- Liver flushes and other natural methods for maintaining liver health
- Hepatitis and cirrhosis, particularly hepatitis C

This book has a four-part format. In the first part, we'll examine what the liver does and how it does it. I have made every effort to make the scientific details understandable to the lay reader. The second part of the book—which may be of more immediate interest to many—presents useful information about what you can actually do to maintain liver health. In the third part, I describe diagnostic signs and symptoms, dietary recommendations, and herbal formulas for eight different liver-related disorders. In the final part, I focus specifically on the causative factors, symptoms, and dietary recommendations for hepatitis (with special attention to hepatitis C) and cirrhosis. I sincerely hope this information will benefit you and your loved ones. However, one word of caution: Though I encourage independent experimentation, I also recommend that you seek the advice of a qualified natural health practitioner for difficult or long-standing liver problems. In any case, good luck on your healing journey!

one

How the Liver Works

THE LIVER'S JOB AND JOB STRESS

The liver's job, in a nutshell, is to make sure that the body absorbs everything it needs and dumps everything it doesn't need. If one were to write a sort of job description for the liver, its list of major duties would look like this:

- Metabolizes proteins, fats, and carbohydrates, thus providing energy and nutrients
- Stores fuel in the form of glycogen, which is especially important to your brain function, and can supply "quick energy"
- Metabolizes drugs and breaks down alcohol

- Stores vitamins, minerals, and sugars
- Filters the blood and helps remove harmful chemicals and bacteria
- Creates bile, which breaks down fats
- Regulates the body's ability to clot
- Governs the transport of fat stores
- Helps assimilate and store fat-soluble vitamins (A, E, D, K); stores iron
- Stores extra blood, which can be quickly released when needed
- Creates serum proteins, which maintain fluid balance and act as carriers for hormones like estrogen and other substances
- Helps maintain electrolyte and water balance
- Creates immune substances, such as gamma globulin
- Regulates levels of sexual hormones: Manufactures estrogen, testosterone, and breaks down and eliminates excess sexual hormones

As you can see, that's a lot of work for a single organ to do even under the best of conditions. Unfortunately, our modern lifestyle burdens the liver with many stresses, making its job even more difficult.

After the insult of oily, processed foods, one of the major stress factors the liver must contend with today is man-made chemicals, such as lead from gasoline, countless food additives, preservatives, pesticides, herbicides, and many other new compounds. It is estimated that chemical companies, in their search for marketable compounds, produce hundreds of new chemicals every year. Since these compounds are completely new to the environment, it may be thousands of years before our bodies evolve and adapt to them.

Other common liver stress factors are alcohol and recreational drugs. Current figures estimate that there are 15.1 million alcoholics and 22 million drug abusers in this country. Furthermore, since drugs administered for therapeutic purposes also affect the liver, 5 percent of hospital patients in the United States (1.9 million people) develop significant adverse reactions to drugs administered by doctors. In fact, 2–4 percent of all hospital admissions (760,000–1.5 million people) are for doctor-prescribed drug reactions.

A final stress our livers must contend with is excess hormones, such as adrenaline, which are constantly being created in our bodies in response to our fast-paced modern lifestyle. Under some circumstances, hormones can be stored by the liver for up to a year, adding fuel to emotional imbalances such as depression and anger as well as to stress-related imbalances such as immune-system depression.

THE LIVER AND DETOXIFICATION

So how exactly does the liver detoxify all the potentially harmful substances that are either put into or created in the body? In order to understand this, we must understand some basic chemistry. Many of the foreign and toxic chemicals that enter the body (either by descending through the food chain into the food we eat or by direct intake of contaminants) are called *lipid soluble*. This means they dissolve only in fatty or oily solutions, not in water. Lipid-soluble compounds have a special affinity for fat tissues and many other cells of the body which have lipid-soluble membranes, such as liver cells. These cells and tissues can store toxins for months, even years, releasing them during times of low food intake, exercise, or stress. As toxins are released, one may experience unpleasant symptoms such as fatigue, dizziness, nausea, or racing pulse.

It is the liver's job to transform lipid-soluble chemicals into water-soluble compounds so that they can be released via the kidneys and bowels. This transformation is carried out by a complex system of enzymes that are made in the *hepatocytes,* or liver cells.

In addition to a complex system of enzymes that remove toxic compounds from the blood, the liver also has filtering channels, called *sinusoids,* that are lined with special cells which engulf and break down foreign debris, bacteria, and toxic chemicals (a process called *phagocytosis*). However, when the liver is burdened with high levels of toxic chemicals or pathogenic organisms (such as *Candida albicans,* a major factor in yeast infections), not all of these substances can be processed and eliminated. In fact, many will be stored in the liver, eventually causing irreparable damage.

As you can see, in natural healing, the liver is considered to be a vital organ in maintaining clean blood, because it actually does act as a blood filter. Many herbalists call certain herbs good "blood purifiers." Does this mean these herbs literally scrub the blood clean? Not really. What actually happens is that the herbs stimulate increased blood flow through the liver, which in turn removes debris, old cells, toxins, etc. At the same time, they protect and stimulate the liver cells, thus encouraging the production of enzymes, which helps to maintain a proper biochemical environment.

Of course, the liver is not the only organ involved in detoxification. Blood purification also depends upon the proper functioning of all the eliminative organs in the body. The skin, for instance, eliminates large quantities of toxins through sweating. That's why sweating therapy and increased fluid intake can often take a load off the liver. Finally, blood purifiers activate such mechanisms of the immune system as the *macrophages* ("big eaters"), which also help remove undesirable elements from the blood.

VITAMINS

Vitamins, minerals, and enzymes are vital to cellular health. They are the "messengers" and "currency" that help make things happen, from the creation of new cells to the production of sexual hormones to the release of energy. Significantly, the liver stores vitamins and minerals for times when they would otherwise be lacking. It can store enough vitamin A to supply an adult's needs for up to four years and enough vitamin D and vitamin B-12 to last for four months!

BILE

The liver also creates bile, which helps break down fats by emulsifying them. Emulsification is the process in which large fat globules are transformed into tiny ones that are more water soluble and easier to assimilate (incidentally, this is the same process by which detergent cleans grimy, oily clothes). To help the liver with this process, a moderate walk after a meal rich in fat is beneficial.

Exercise encourages the fat to move through the body and facilitates its processing.

Excessive amounts of fat and protein in the diet are difficult for the liver to break down because they make the liver work harder to produce bile and other digestive enzymes. In addition, ammonia produced by the metabolic breakdown of protein can irritate or even be toxic to the liver. Thus, when the liver is not functioning properly, or if it is diseased, it is important to eat fewer foods that contain fat and protein, such as meat and dairy products. It is also good to eat more easily assimilated complex carbohydrates, such as rice or millet, because these take a great load off the liver by decreasing the amount of bile needed. This will also help to build up and better utilize glycogen (the storage form of glucose) in the hepatocytes, which means the liver will have more energy to rebuild itself and establish proper harmony.

One major cause of impaired bile flow is gallstones. Current medical literature states that at least 20 million people in the United States have gallstones. Bile stagnation can also result from actual cellular damage to the liver due to the negative effects of alcohol, hyperthyroidism or thyroxine supplementation, exposure to toxic drugs or other synthetic chemicals, and the use of birth control pills. When the bile is stagnant, the skin becomes sallow, yellow, or blemished. Also, important vitamins are not assimilated properly, which can impair blood clotting, vision, and the body's antioxidant system. Further damage to the body may occur when toxic compounds that are usually cycled through the bile and eliminated are held in the liver instead.

Many ancient systems of healing recognized the fact that bile is a vital bodily fluid. Throughout the world herbs are commonly taken to restore proper bile flow, for when the bile is stagnant, sadness and disharmony can result. The word *melancholy,* for instance, comes from the Greek *melanos* ("black") and *chole* ("bile"), or literally "black bile." This condition has been called "sluggish liver" in Western medicine and "liver stagnation" in Traditional Chinese Medicine (TCM).

ENZYMES

An enzyme is a complex protein that speeds up a chemical reaction in the body. Many (indeed most) of the chemical reactions that are going on inside us every second would not occur naturally unless the various reactants were heated to high temperatures. That is because the reactions of life generally require a great deal of energy in order to take place. However, enzymes allow these critical reactions to occur at body temperature. Each enzyme (there are thousands of different kinds!) has its own, unique shape that allows it to "fit" with only certain molecules, like pieces of a jigsaw puzzle. When an enzyme attaches to its matching molecule, it can help break it into smaller pieces, or it can "glue" many smaller molecules together into a larger one. Thus enzymes speed up the chemical reactions involved in both the building up and breaking down (*digestion*) of substances in the body.

As we have already seen, during the detoxification process the liver makes use of various enzymes. Actually, these are not individual enzymes but whole enzyme systems, referred to collectively as the Microsomal Enzyme System (MES). The MES is part of our evolutionary legacy. Its job is to process many different kinds of chemicals, as already explained. Most likely, the liver developed these enzyme systems to deactivate, and facilitate the elimination of, naturally occurring *endogenous* (produced within the body) chemicals such as bilirubin, serotonin, and the hormones estradiol and testosterone. The MES probably also evolved to help detoxify and eliminate many natural toxins present in the wild and in slightly spoiled foods, which were common before the advent of refrigeration.

Although the MES is necessary for survival, it is something of a double-edged sword. On the one hand, it can transform fat-soluble toxic chemicals, such as DDT, into more water-soluble ones that are easily eliminated via the bowels and urine. On the other hand, ironically, the MES can also transform certain nontoxic compounds into toxic or even carcinogenic ones. For example, toxic alkaloids found in the medicinal plant comfrey are probably harmless until they travel through the liver and are transformed into highly potent compounds that can lead to liver damage (hence both researchers and herbalists now recommend caution in the use of comfrey products, especially during pregnancy).

The different kinds of enzyme systems in the MES have been classified into two types: phase I and phase II systems. Phase I systems alter chemical groups on the foreign substances, rendering them more water soluble and hence disposable. Phase II systems, in contrast, generally help to conjugate (or bind) compounds with sulfur-containing groups, presumably to make them less toxic or, as in the case of bodily hormones, to deactivate them.

Every cell in the body contains sulfur compounds, which are vital to their health and proper functioning. Glutathione is an important sulfur-containing compound the body produces. It is one of the most potent free-radical scavengers in the body, helping to protect cells from damage resulting from these highly reactive molecules produced after exposure to noxious chemicals or immune activation. The liver produces glutatione, which also aids the liver in the breakdown of many damaging substances such as pesticides or industrial chemicals in our water or food. Such liver stressors as alcohol consumption or viral infections always lead to glutathione depletion, which reduces the liver's ability to protect itself against the harmful effects of many of the noxious agents it has to detoxify.

Most Phase I reactions are facilitated by enzymes known as mixed-function oxidases (MFO), the most common of which is the Cytochrome P-450 system. Cytochrome P-450 plays a central role in detoxifying numerous potentially hazardous compounds. It also assists in the synthesis of steroid hormones and, with vitamin C, works in an important step of bile synthesis. Unfortunately for the liver, however, certain toxic chemicals disrupt the P-450 system. These toxic chemicals include common herbicides and pesticides, as well as breakdown products from them that can linger in the environment for many years (for instance DDE, a breakdown product from DDT, is still abundant in the environment many years after DDT was banned). These can be stored in fat tissues and slowly released into the bloodstream, eventually finding their way to the liver. Because the production of synthetic pesticides exceeds 1.4 billion pounds a year in the United States, it is likely that there are enough toxic substances in the environment to adversely affect our livers and lives.

Phase II systems, for their part, include both UDP-glucuronyl transferase (GT), and glutathione-S-transferase (GSH-T). Glutathione (GSH-T) is one of the most important endogenous antioxidants and cellular protectors in the body. It can be depleted by large amounts of drugs or toxic chemicals passing through the liver, as well as by fasting or starvation. GSH-T is also subject to circadian rhythms, which means that its levels increase and decrease according to the body's twenty-four-hour biological cycles. Thus there is 30 percent less GSH-T in the body in the late afternoon than late at night.

So what does all this mean for our health? Well, while natural amounts of substances such as GT and GSH-T are vital to optimal liver function, excessive amounts may be harmful. High GSH-T levels in the liver can cause the transformation of nontoxic chemicals into more toxic ones that damage the liver. Thus, there must be just enough GHS-T available for important enzymatic reactions, but not so much as to cause excessive transformations. In other words, health depends upon biochemical tone. Tone means that there is just enough of a particular substance, action, or force to maintain a state of dynamic equilibrium in the body and consequently the ability to function. The Chinese call this the balance of yin and yang, but many Westerners prefer the concept of tone. Some simple but effective ways to maintain proper tone in the GSH-T and the liver's other enzyme systems include exercise, positive attitude, visualization, polarity therapy, and various other common methods for bringing about greater health, such as a balanced diet and ample water intake. Also, we can use herbs and other dietary measures, which we shall soon address in depth.

THE LIVER AND EMOTIONAL BALANCE

In the preceding pages we have discussed several technical and scientific concepts. How do these relate to the everyday lives of thinking, feeling human beings? Well, most important is the fact that any emotions a person feels have a basis in biochemistry. When you feel angry, for instance, a complex mixture of hormones and other chemicals speeds to various parts of your body, readying you for action. Likewise, fear, jealousy, joy, sorrow, and all our other emotions have a corresponding chemical reality which can create profound changes in our bodies. And depending on the strength and duration of the emotions, these changes can more or less determine a person's character and outlook on life.

Thus, an important function of the liver, which is just now beginning to be understood, is its role in transforming and removing excess hormones from the blood. When the liver is diseased or functioning poorly, its ability to do this is impaired. Then emotional states that should come and go easily linger far longer than necessary. An environment full of negative or excessive emotions burdens the liver.

Take anger, for instance. According to TCM, anger is associated with the liver and gallbladder. (Westerners would say that the bile in the gallbladder can store the excess hormones not eliminated by a poorly functioning liver.) Similarly, in Ayurvedic medicine anger is associated with the fire principle and the liver. Thus in either case someone who is chronically angry would be said to have an unhealthy liver or gallbladder. The prescribed treatment would be gentle opening, cleansing, and perhaps cooling of the bile and liver, using herbs and liver flushes (all of which will be discussed in detail later).

THE LIVER AND PMS

Having understood this much about the liver and emotions, it should be easy to grasp their connection with premenstrual syndrome (PMS). More than 40 million women in the United States alone suffer from symptoms related to PMS, and more than 5 million require some form of medical treatment.

Although all the causes of PMS are not known, it is likely that excess estrogen, a steroid hormone, plays an important role. Estrogen is known to rise just after menstruation, peaking about mid-cycle during ovulation. It then drops, slowly rises again, and falls a second time just before the onset of menstruation. Fluid retention contributing to water-weight gain and mood changes has been directly linked to increased estrogen.

Again, it is the liver's job to clear away any excess estrogen circulating through the body. However, if the body produces too much estrogen, the liver may not be able to keep up with its job, resulting in PMS symptoms such as depression, cramps, headaches, fatigue, or even more serious problems. For instance, excess estrogen has been reported to increase the risk of gallbladder disease; production of clots and inflammation in the blood vessels; high blood pressure; hyperglycemia; and breast, uterine, liver, and vaginal cancer. Current research is emphasizing that circulating estrogen levels in both men and women may be increased by environmental and dietary factors such as electromagnetic radiation (from appliances, power lines, etc.), PCBs from electrical equipment, herbicides and pesticides such as DDT, and alcohol consumption.

Fortunately, natural therapy can help your liver with all types of hormonal imbalances, including PMS. For women who do not produce enough estrogen and consequently receive prescribed estrogen therapy (as well as for those who suffer from osteoporosis and symptoms associated with menopause), it is especially important to support the liver with natural therapy. For those who suffer from emotional swings, food cravings, and other undesirable symptoms caused by estrogen excess, natural plant remedies can partially block the binding sites estrogen normally uses to activate or modify cellular processes in estrogen-sensitive tissue. In this way, natural plant remedies can prevent estrogen from overextending the scope and amount of its beneficial activities.

Besides estrogen, testosterone, too, is metabolized by the liver. Testosterone, which exists in both the male and female body, is known to affect levels of aggressiveness and sexual en-

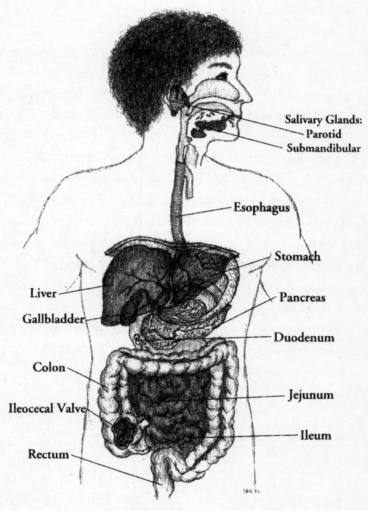

The Human Digestive Tract

ergy. Hence if the liver cannot properly eliminate excess testosterone, overly aggressive behavior, extreme mood swings, and abnormal levels of sexual energy may result, as well as dysfunction of the reproductive cycle.

THE CHINESE LIVER SYSTEM

So far we have discussed the liver as it is known to Western science. The concept of the liver in TCM is somewhat different and merits closer study. My TCM teacher told me that nothing escapes yin-yang theory, meaning that according to Chinese culture, everything in the material universe is an interaction of two opposing forces. Everything in the known universe has two aspects that are constantly interacting, changing, and blending into one another. One cannot exist without the other; in fact, they are different aspects of the same thing. Health is created in the body when yin and yang are in harmony or balance. As soon as this balance is disrupted, disease results. The concept of yin and yang is profound and pervasive. Although Westerners don't necessarily think in these terms, once you examine carefully this universal concept and begin to understand it, you will find new ways to look at health and disease and how they are created, destroyed, or maintained.

Yin	Yang
Matter	Energy
Rest (passive)	Recuperation (active)
Vital substance	Vital function

Yin is created from yang. Yang arises from yin. Too much metabolic activity results in the depletion of yin and an excess of yang.

Too little metabolic activity results in a deficiency of yang and the accumulation of yin.

The ancient healing system of TCM recognizes five bodily systems, each of which is associated with one of the five primary elements in nature. Also, each of the principal internal organs is thought to be connected to an external part of the body which it affects, to an external anatomical part where the condition of the internal organ is reflected, and to an emotion and climatic condition. Table 1 summarizes these basic relationships.

TABLE 1

The Fundamental Relationships of TCM

Organ System	Element	Diagnostic Part	Affected Parts	Climate	Taste	Emotions
Stomach/ spleen	Earth	Mouth	Flesh/lips	Moisture	Sweet	Worry
Lungs/ colon	Metal	Nasal cavities	Skin/body hair	Dryness	Acrid	Grief/ despair
Kidney/ bladder	Water	Ears/head/ hair	Bones	Coldness	Salty	Fear/ anxiety
Liver/ gallbladder	Wood	Eyes	Tendons/ nails/ ligaments	Wind	Sour	Anger/ irritability
Heart/ pericardium/ Small intestine	Fire	Tongue	Vascular system/ complexion	Heat	Bitter	Joy/ mania

According to TCM, the liver's main job is to regulate the flow of qi (pronounced "chee," meaning, approximately, "life energy" or "vital energy"). Qi is responsible for all activity of the body, the blood, the qi itself, and for proper functioning of the organs. The liver moves the blood and qi smoothly in all directions throughout the body and harmonizes the functioning of the organs. Naturally, then, the liver is particularly sensitive to anything that disrupts what the Chinese so aptly call its "free and easy wanderer" movement and influence within the body. Excessive or negative emotions, especially, will disrupt this free-flowing ambience, causing deficiency, coldness, or stagnation. The net result of any such blockage of energy in the liver is a buildup of toxins, which can cause cellular damage and poor functioning of the Microsomal Enzyme System (MES) discussed earlier. This in turn may lead to further damage from free radicals and peroxidized lipids, which we shall address later.

As well as being susceptible to blockage or qi stagnation, the liver is also susceptible to overstimulation. In the latter condition, the liver receives too much blood and goes into a sort of metabolic overdrive called "blazing fire" in TCM. This state can be caused by alcohol, drugs, and an excess of certain spices, such as black pepper. Blazing fire can remain localized in the liver and cause overheating, which in Western terms may lead to enzyme dysfunction and damage to the hepatocytes. This syndrome approximates some forms of hepatitis or cirrhosis. Or the heat can rise up to the head, inducing headaches, facial flushing, thirst, dizziness, and ringing in the ears.

In addition to regulating the flow of chi in the body, the liver has other important functions in TCM. First, it regulates digestive activity. When the liver fails in this task because of a loss of biochemical harmony, its action can "invade," or negatively affect, the stomach, thus precipitating digestive problems such as abdominal pain, nausea, burping, and diarrhea.

Second, in TCM just as in Western medicine, the liver also controls the bile. If the bile does not flow smoothly, jaundice, loss of appetite, and a bitter taste in the mouth will result. Fats will not be well tolerated or assimilated, and the fat-soluble vitamins A, E, D, and K will not be utilized well—a situation that can lead to immune system depression.

Third, the liver harmonizes the emotions. According to some TCM texts, it has a "sprinkling" movement that is responsible for maintaining a relaxed and flowing inner environment and an even-tempered disposition. This works in a cyclic way: A healthy liver helps maintain an even temperament and vice versa. However, if the cycle turns downward, a turbulent emotional climate can damage the liver, and the injured liver will further aggravate the emotional chaos.

Fourth, an important function of the liver, understood by TCM and Western medicine alike, is the storage of extra blood for use in times of need, as during physical activity. However, according to TCM, imbalances occur if the liver either does not have enough extra blood stored (resulting in dryness in the eyes), or loses its ability to store blood properly (resulting in excessive menstrual flow). The liver is also thought to regulate the blood, which is not surprising, since the blood and qi work together in the body.

Last, it is important to note that TCM texts state that the liver also "rules" the tendons and is manifested in the nails. This can provide helpful diagnostic information. For example, if the tendons are stiff, hard, and painful, or weak, with increased susceptibility to injury, or if the nails are pale and brittle, then it could mean that the liver is failing to nourish them properly.

Remember that in TCM all these aspects of liver functioning are interrelated, so that in reality no one aspect can be separated from the others. We only look at them separately because this helps us to draw conclusions about functional disharmony and successful treatment.

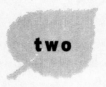

two

Natural Therapy for the Liver

GENERAL DIETARY GUIDELINES

Now that we have a fairly good idea of how the liver does its work, let's take a look at what a person can do to maintain optimum liver health. First we'll discuss dietary factors and practices that everyone should consider. Even if you aren't suffering from any obvious liver disorder at the moment, good eating habits can save you from developing problems later. After examining diet, we'll then address herbal therapies for a variety of liver-related disorders and imbalances. We are now in the "practical" section of this book, so this information is useless unless you actually APPLY it!

First of all, here is an overview of signs and symptoms to help you determine if your liver system is under stress or not functioning properly:

- Frequent headaches not related to tension and stress in the neck and shoulders (from poor posture when sitting and studying, for instance) or to eye strain
- Ongoing menstrual problems
- Weak tendons, ligaments, and muscles
- Acne, psoriasis, and other skin problems
- Tenderness or pain in the liver area
- Emotional excess, especially anger and depression; moodiness
- Blurring of vision or red eyes
- Bitter taste in the mouth

If you experience any of these symptoms, I recommend that you consult with a trained holistic health practitioner and receive a comprehensive dietary, lifestyle, and herbal program, though if symptoms are mild, self-treatment is often appropriate.

FATS AND OILS

One of the greatest dangers in the modern diet is the kinds and quantities of fats and oils it contains. This is particularly pertinent to the liver, as it is a major site where fats and oils accumulate and are processed. Recently, people have started to eat more unsaturated fats because of the bad press saturated fats have received concerning their role in heart disease, a major killer in industrial countries. Ironically, however, manufacturers are now touting foods containing only unsaturated fats as being healthy and natural when the truth may be, in switching from saturated to unsaturated fats, we are only trading heart disease for cancer, premature aging, excessive skin wrinkles, and liver damage.

How so? Well, it all relates to how oxygen affects fats and oils in the body. Oxygen is the key element in the basic metabolic process of *oxidation,* that is, the burning up and breaking down of nutrients and other molecules. Many of the body's chemical reactions depend on oxygen as a sort of catalytic fuel. However, because oxygen is a very reactive element, it doesn't always stick to only helpful biochemical reactions; it can also create harmful reactions by oxidizing various susceptible substances. Unsaturated oils are highly prone to such dangerous oxidation because of their carbon-carbon double bonds, which are easily attacked by oxygen.

Oil that has been oxidized becomes rancid. It should never be eaten because doing so can lead to the creation of free radicals in the body. Free radicals are molecules or unstable atoms, like oxygen, with an unpaired electron that makes them highly reactive to certain parts of healthy cells, such as cell-wall components and even DNA. Modern medical researchers think that free radicals "attack" the body's cells and lead to widespread tissue damage (such as in the liver), thus accelerating the aging process. Indeed, there is a free-radical theory of aging, which proposes that many signs of aging, such as loss of flexibility and function in the joints, skin, and even internal organs (especially the liver), are promoted by free radicals.

Now about 17 percent of our total oxygen consumption turns into free radicals that can damage lipids and other cellular molecules. Most oxygen-consuming organisms have evolved defense systems to keep such free-radical damage to tolerable levels. In human beings, these natural defense mechanisms include enzyme systems, such as the glutathione (GSH-T) peroxidase system we discussed earlier; naturally occurring antioxidants such as vitamin C, A, and especially E; and DNA repair mechanisms. Nonetheless, these natural defense mechanisms did not evolve with the modern diet in mind, so they may need to be supplemented with healing plants that provide many of the essential elements needed to sustain them.

Having said this much about the underpublicized dangers of unsaturated oil, I must turn around and emphasize that unsaturated oils are not all bad. On the contrary, highly unsaturated fatty acids (such as linoleic acid), are crucial to human health—in moderate doses and preferably unheated. If you avoid junk and snack foods, eat a diet rich in whole, unprocessed foods, and take herbs and/or other supplements that contain antioxidants, you are in no danger of getting too much unsaturated oil.

Here are some general recommendations regarding oils and fats:

- Olive oil (extra virgin), the most natural to our bodies, is resistant to oxidation and contains a good balance of saturated, monosaturated (oleic), and unsaturated fatty acids (linoleic and linolenic). Oleic acid is less affected by oxygen and has been shown in a number of recent studies to benefit the heart and cardiovascular system.
- Flaxseed oil provides a rich source of essential fatty, linoleic, and linolenic acids.
- Avoid margarine, which contains oils that have been heated and pressurized to change their molecular structure—a biochemical nightmare for the body, especially for the liver.

- Lightly salted raw butter is superior to margarine. Where no refrigeration is available, ghee (clarified butter) can be used because it won't spoil, which is why it is eaten in India.
- Unsaturated oils, such as sunflower and safflower, should be tasted for rancidity (a sharp, biting taste). They should be stored in the refrigerator once opened.
- As much as possible, obtain essential fatty acids and other oils the body needs from whole nuts and seeds, preferably raw and organically grown. I prefer almonds and walnuts raw and unheated. Almonds can be soaked overnight and blended after soaking to make almond milk for easier digestibility.

Table 2 gives the percentage composition of saturated and unsaturated fatty acids in several common nuts, seeds, fats, and oils.

BITTER TONICS, OR "BITTERS"

In the traditional medicine of both Europe and China, bitter herbs are thought to tonify and strengthen the digestive, immune, and nervous systems. Bitter tonic formulas, often called "bitters," usually contain bitter herbs like gentian, goldenseal, artichoke, angelica, or blessed thistle, plus some aromatic or spicy herbs (ginger, fennel, or cardamom) to help counteract the formula's ability to cool and contract the digestive tract in some people. Many ready-made bitter formulas are available in natural-food stores and in some grocery stores and liquor stores (angostura bitters), though when they come from the latter two

TABLE 2

Fatty Acid Composition of Common
Nuts, Seeds, Fats, and Oils

Source	Total Fat (gms of fat per 100 gms)	Saturated Fat, %	Oleic Acid, %	Total Unsaturated Fat, %
Nuts, seeds				
Almonds	54.2	8	67	19
Brazil nuts	66.9	26	33	38
Cashew nuts	45.7	20	57	17
Filberts	62.4	7	80	11
Peanuts	48.7	17	48	24
Sunflower seeds	47.3	13	19	64
Walnuts, English	64.0	11	15	66
Fats, Oils				
Butter	81	62	25	4
Corn oil	100	17	24	59
Cottonseed oil	100	26	18	52
Flaxseed oil	100	9	19	72
Lard	100	40	41	15
Olive oil	100	16	76	8
Palm kernel oil	100	85	13	2
Peanut oil	100	18	47	29
Rapeseed (canola) oil	100	7	50	37
Sesame oil	100	13	42	45
Soybean oil	100	15	26	59
Fish				
Salmon	7.4	18	18	39

sources they must be checked for sugar, preservatives, and other undesirable additives.

Bitters are still used extensively in many cultures to strengthen digestion. In Europe, for example, "bitters cafés" are a popular social stop on the way home from work to prime the digestive tract for the evening meal. European naturopaths regularly recommend bitter wild greens or small doses of unripe fruit (such as green apples) to increase digestive powers. When I traveled in Greece years ago, I was delighted to discover that people there customarily eat small, unripe, sour and bitter plums before meals. The Greeks also like to begin major meals with wild chicory greens, which are known to contain mild bitter principles that activate the digestive juices.

The traditional use of bitters makes good scientific sense, since by reflexive nerve action the bitter flavor immediately activates the secretion of gastric juices and tonifies the muscles of the digestive tract. Research has shown that bitters also activate the parasympathetic nervous system (which "controls" the digestive tract) as well as the immune system. Indeed, some bitter compounds, such as the amarogentin in the herb gentian, are so powerfully bitter that they can be detected in a dilution of 1:50,000!

How to Take Bitters

It is important to understand that bitters must be taken over a period of weeks before their full effect is achieved. Taking them for a day or two might bestow some benefits, but 90 percent of the effect is cumulative.

Bitter formulas are taken 15–30 minutes before a meal, or just after eating. Take ½ to 1 teaspoon of the liquid extract; 1–2 teaspoons of a bitters tea (at room temperature, not hot); or 1 dropperful of a more concentrated formula. Note that some commercial bitters also contain a mild laxative herb such as aloe or senna. These should be avoided by people who have diarrhea or loose bowels. I have also found that these formulas may not agree with people who lack vital energy and who are often fatigued.

Here's a recipe for making homemade bitters.

Artichoke (1 part)   Cardamon (¼ part)
Gentian (¼ part)   Ginger rhizome (¼ part)
Orange or tangerine peel (1 part)

Powder the dried herbs in a blender and add to either vodka or wine. Macerate the mixture (i.e., let it soak) for 1–2 weeks, shaking the jar every day. Press or squeeze out the liquid and then filter (optional). Store in suitable clean glass containers or amber dropper bottles (available in drug stores).

To make bitters tea, simmer 1 part herb mixture to 20 parts water for 30 minutes.

NOTE: This tea cannot be kept outside the refrigerator without fermenting, and even in the refrigerator, it should not be kept for more than 3 days.

OTHER DIETARY FACTORS

The following is a short list of other dietary factors to consider when you are trying to eat for optimal liver health. Table 3 summarizes handy dietary sources of substances that build, protect, and/or cleanse the liver.

• Deciding how to eat for a healthy liver is actually a no-brainer. The less industrial processing your food undergoes the better. The less added fat and sugar your food contains the better. Avoid fried foods, especially meats. Eat the highest quality organic food, preferably straight from the garden.

Warming your food, especially in cold climates, can be good, but avoid overcooking vegetables. They should remain slightly crunchy.

• Protein: Both too little or too much can disrupt liver enzymes. About 35–60 grams per day is optimal. Most people in industrialized countries eat far too much protein. When bacteria in the large intestine act on protein residues, toxins that may be absorbed into the bloodstream are produced. Good sources of protein include fish, occasional organic meat (if desired), nuts, seeds, beans and grains, and nutritional yeast.

• Sulfur-containing foods such as cabbage, Brussels sprouts, broccoli, nuts, and seeds are potent enzyme builders. Have at least one serving a day of these foods, especially vegetables from the mustard family, which provide excellent enzyme support for the liver.

• Fats are difficult for the liver to process, yet they provide a good energy source. A small amount of unsaturated fat is essential to health, but an excess will oxidize easily, leading to the formation of potentially harmful free radicals. A variety of raw, organic nuts, seeds, grains, beans, and, if you desire, fish, can supply the best-quality oils.

• Vitamins, minerals, herbs, amino acids, and flavonoids protect the liver and should be present in ample amounts. To make sure you are getting enough, I recommend live vegetable juices (carrot, beet, celery, or parsley). Or, if you don't have the time or incentive to make juice, perhaps take a complete nutritional system supplement to insure you are getting everything your body needs.

• Refined sugars, such as glucose, can lower enzyme activity. Sweet foods can be a healthful addition to the diet if they contain predominantly complex and unrefined sugars, such as those found in all fruits, vegetables, whole grains, and in barley malt and rice syrup. For a sweeter treat, use more concentrated sugars such as dates, dried fruit, pure unrefined cane sugar, and honey in moderation.

• Phosphatidyl choline is a constituent of lecithin that can improve the health of the microsomal membrane (in the liver) where enzymes are produced. Soybean products are a good source of this substance, as is commercially available lecithin.

TABLE 3
Dietary Sources of Liver Builders, Cleansers, and Protectors

Substance Type	Source	Constituents
Antioxidants	whole seeds	vitamin E
	fruit	vitamin C
	green or red peppers	carotenoids
	brightly colored vegetables and their juice	carotenoids, flavonoids
	sprouts	vitamin C
	spirulina	superoxide dismutase
Cleansers	fruits	citric acid, pectin
		raw vegetable juices
Builders	seeds, nuts	protein, fatty acids, minerals
		(iron, vitamin B-rich foods)
Protectors	cole crops (cabbage, broccoli, etc.)	organic sulfur compounds
Enzyme builders	cole crops, other vegetables	vitamins, organic sulfur compounds

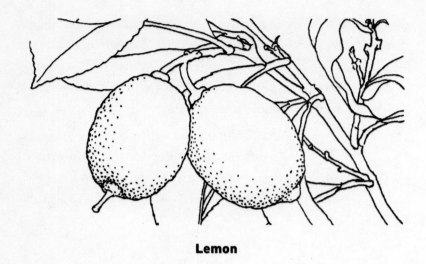

Lemon

Citrus limon

THE LIVER FLUSH

Liver flushes are used to stimulate elimination of wastes from the body, to open and cool the liver, to increase bile flow, and to improve overall liver functioning. They also help purify the blood and the lymph. I have taken liver flushes for many years now and can heartily recommend them. And if you make the herbal formula right, it can be quite tasty. Here's how to make a liver flush:

1. Mix any freshly squeezed citrus juices to make 1 cup of liquid. Orange and grapefruit juices are good, but always mix in some lemon or lime. The final mix should have a tart taste—the more sour, the more cleansing and activating. This mixture can be watered down to taste with spring or distilled water.

2. Add 1–2 cloves of freshly squeezed garlic, plus a small amount of fresh ginger juice, which you can obtain by

grating ginger on a cheese or vegetable grater and then pressing the resulting fibers in a garlic press. (Note: Both garlic and ginger have been shown to have amazing liver-protecting qualities in recent studies. Garlic contains strong antioxidant principles and also provides important sulfur compounds the liver uses to build certain enzymes.)

3. Mix in 1 tablespoon of high-quality olive oil (preferably extra virgin and organic), blend (or shake well in a glass container), and drink.

4. Follow the liver flush with 2 cups of cleansing herbal tea, which consists of the herbs listed below. I make plenty of this tea and keep it in quart canning jars or juice bottles, so it is always available.

5. Drink the liver flush in the morning (preferably after some stretching and breathing exercises), and do not eat any other food for one hour.

CLEANSING POLARI-TEA

Fennel seed (1 part)

Fenugreek seed (1 part)

Flaxseed (1 part)

Burdock root (½ part)

Licorice root (¼ part)

Peppermint (1 part)

Marshmallow root (1 part),
    cut and sifted (opt.)

Simmer the herbs for 20 minutes, then add 1 part peppermint and let the tea steep for an additional 10 minutes. For extra soothing properties, try adding ½ part marshmallow root (cut and sifted) to the original tea blend.

NOTE: The Polari-Tea tends to have a cooling effect. If you feel hot, or have symptoms or an illness related to heat and you need a cooler formula, add oregon grape root and dandelion root; if you need a "warmer" formula, add ginger and cardamom.

When and how often should one take liver flushes? I usually do two full cycles of 10 days on, 3 days off in the spring and again in the fall, with a 3-day rest between each cycle. However, I know many people who benefit from a single 10-day flush once at each equinox, spring and fall. In any case, though, if you feel a need for a liver flush, any time is the right time. It is rare, but some may experience negative side effects from this procedure, including mild nausea and upset stomach.

There are also several good commercial formulas for liver cleansing available in natural-food stores, both in bulk and in tea-bag form. One product I can recommend is a blend called "Puri-Tea," from herbalist Brigitte Mars. It contains pepper-mint, red clover, fennel, licorice, cleavers, dandelion, Oregon grape, burdock root, butternut bark, chickweed, parsley root, and nettles.

THE GALLBLADDER FLUSH

NOTE: This technique is for people who have had previous experi-ence with cleansing programs and have followed a predomi-nantly whole-foods diet for some time.

The gallbladder flush is useful for people who are experi-enced with fasting and cleansing and who want to go a step fur-ther and remove even more old wastes stored in liver cells and other tissues. This flush should not be used more than once a year. I have seen some people become nauseated after drinking the flush, but nothing worse than that. Of course you may never be able to face salad dressing again ☺.

1. About an hour before bedtime, drink ¼ cup of extra-virgin olive oil, followed by ¼ cup of mixed, freshly squeezed citrus juices (50 percent grapefruit juice, 25 percent lemon juice, and 25 percent orange juice). Repeat this process every 15 minutes for an hour, so that you drink a total of 1 cup of olive oil and 1 cup of citrus juice.
2. After the drinks, go to bed, making sure to lie on your right side. By tradition, this is thought to allow the oil to be discharged from the gallbladder more efficiently, but whether this is in fact true has not been proven as far as I know.
3. In the morning, take an enema consisting of 1 quart of warm distilled water with the addition of the juice of ¼ lemon.

NOTE: It is often good to combine the gallbladder flush with a 3- or 7-day juice fast (see page 32). Toxic wastes released during fasting will be effectively eliminated during the strong bile flush and enema.

The purpose of this flush is to strongly activate the liver and gallbladder. When the liver encounters so much oil, it reacts by producing a large amount of bile, which the gallbladder then squirts into the intestines. It is thought that such a strong flow of bile will carry with it deeply stored toxins which are then flushed out of the body with the enema. Activating the liver and gallbladder so strongly may also run them through a thorough drill, thus offering a kind of "tune-up."

During the enema, watch for little green "stones" or marbles that may be eliminated. I have heard these called gallstones, but they are probably saponified oil. At any rate, my own experience with the flush, plus my observation of others who have done it, have convinced me that old, negative emotions can be effectively eliminated during the process.

Anger and frustration, especially, are purged. It is possible that one may experience strange feelings during the process, as if some drug were floating around in the bloodstream. This may be due to old drug residues being reexperienced as they are eliminated from the body, or it may be due to a systemic hormonal reaction to all the oil. I tend to believe the former theory, but no definitive tests have been conducted to prove which view is right.

If you want more cleansing action than simple teas or formulas provide, try adding a fast with fresh fruit and vegetable juices. You can also take an enema each day. A good enema can be made by adding the juice of ½ lemon to 1 quart of tepid water (lemon-water in general is a good cleanser because citric and other plant acids in lemon juice can chelate [i.e., bind with] and remove heavy metals and other toxic wastes accumulated in the body). Retain for 10–15 minutes (if possible), apply clockwise lower abdominal massage, then expel. For complete cleansing and fasting programs, see *The Miracle of Fasting* by Paul C. Bragg.

THE THREE-DAY JUICE FAST

For a novice faster, I usually recommend a short 3-day fast using fruit juices. Water fasts are often too severe for most people and

TABLE 4

Benefits of Fasting

Cleanses

The body is very wise. When it can't get energy and nutrients from food, it breaks down diseased and second-rate or toxic cells, recycles the usable components, and eliminates wastes.

Allows Rest

Gives your digestive system a much-deserved rest.

Increases Energy

Tremendous amounts of vital energy usually spent in digestion, assimilation, and elimination are saved for other purposes.

Promotes Weight Loss

Not eating is the fastest way to lose excess weight. Fat is broken down before muscle tissue in the fasting process.

Heals

Even intractable diseases have been healed during fasts.

Breaks Addictions

Fasting is one of the very best ways to break addictions. It can strengthen discrimination and willpower. After a fast, the last thing you want to do is smoke a cigarette or drink coffee or alcohol. Many years ago, I broke a seemingly unbreakable addiction to tobacco with a fast.

Saves Time

Hours a day are often spent in working to pay for food, shopping, preparing food, eating, and cleaning up the kitchen.

Restores Appreciation

In no period of human history has such a variety of food been as readily available as today. There is so much abundance that it is easy to become blasé about delicacies such as tropical fruits and artichoke hearts. Fasting helps us realize just how blessed we really are. I still vividly remember how delicious a bite of apple tasted after my first 2-week fast. The finest ambrosia of the goddesses and gods couldn't be better.

---

are not the best kind of fast for the industrial chemicals and heavy metals that may be stored in our bodies these days. Besides, fruit juices contain pectin, fruit acids, and other purifying substances that help remove toxic wastes.

Always eat raw fruits and vegetables for two or three days before and after the fast, to ease in and out of the fasting period. During the fast, drink nothing but water and freshly extracted juices. If fresh juice is impossible to obtain during the fast, then use bottled organic grape or apple juice diluted in a 1:1 ratio with distilled water. However, even freshly squeezed grapefruit juice and distilled water is preferable to bottled juices because the body responds best to the vitality of fresh juice. Note that the whole process actually lasts 10 days, counting preparation and transition to a normal diet.

The Program

Days 1–3 (Preparations): Upon rising, do 20–40 minutes of deep breathing and stretching (such as yoga) and continue this every day throughout the fast. Then drink a liver flush (detailed on page 28). Follow with 2 cups of cleansing tea. Eat raw fruits and vegetables, salads, whole apples, pears, grapefruit—but not bananas (juicy foods only).

Drink as much distilled water with fresh lemon juice added to taste as desired. More herbal tea in the evening is optional.

Days 4–6 (The Fast): Start each day during the actual fast with the liver flush and tea, and follow one or two hours later with about 6–8 ounces of freshly squeezed fruit juice (usually apple, grape, or grapefruit) diluted with distilled water in a 1:1 ratio. A few hours later, try 6–8 ounces of mixed vegetable juice, usually a combination of organic carrot and celery, with a touch of beet or parsley. In the evening take another glass of fruit juice and perhaps a cup of herb tea. Finally, before bed take an enema consisting of 1 quart of warm distilled water mixed with the juice of ½ lemon. If you've never taken an enema before, you may be surprised at how much comes out. During a fast the bowels will usually cease to move. The enema will remove waste material that is being eliminated into the colon and will also soften and remove old fecal matter that may be hanging onto the walls of the colon. Make sure to drink plenty of distilled water or other high-quality water, at least a quart or two with the addition of the juice of 1 lemon per quart of water.

Day 6 or 7 (the last day of the fast): I usually go to a professional for a colonic flush. This ensures that my colon is thoroughly cleaned. During the colonic, I am always amazed at what I see come out—even after fasting and taking enemas. Some people prefer to have a series of two or three colonics after a fast, but my feeling is that one is enough.

Day 8: I always break a 3-day fast with a raw salad (see Paul Bragg's *The Miracle of Fasting*). I have tried different ways to break a short fast and have found this to be the most satisfactory. The roughage in the salad helps move the bowels and acts as a sort of "broom" to sweep out additional wastes. My first salad consists of grated cabbage, carrot, finely chopped celery, a little grated beet root, and perhaps some finely shredded romaine lettuce. I eat a good-sized bowl of this salad at about noon of the day after the 3-day fast (the eighth day overall). In the evening I eat more raw vegetables, or a little vegetable broth, depending on how I am feeling.

Day 9: Eat fruits and vegetables during the day, with the addition of a steamed potato or other steamed green vegetables.

Day 10: Begin to eat regularly, but lightly. Chew each bite well and combine foods carefully. I always find that by this time I desire no processed foods. It feels so good to have had the discipline and wisdom to fast that I don't want to put anything in my body that is not the very best fresh, organic food.

Side Effects

I have never seen any serious problems during a fast, but it is common to experience symptoms such as:

- Dizziness
- Mild heart palpitations
- Weakness
- Light-headedness
- Fatigue
- Forgetfulness
- Mild nausea
- A bad taste in the mouth, known as "faster's breath"
- A gnawing or empty feeling in the stomach and abdomen

I recommend consulting a natural health-care practitioner, such as a naturopathic physician, who has experience supervising fasts if you are feeling weak or run-down, have a serious heart condition or any medical condition that requires medication, or you are pregnant or nursing.

If the usual side effects of the fast become unpleasant, you can slow down the cleansing process by using a juice or broth that is less cleansing for a short time, until the symptoms abate. Also, it always helps to rest, if possible, and to focus on the positive aspects of the cleansing and healing process. Envision the wastes leaving your body. I often imagine a pure mountain meadow filled with wildflowers and with a crystal clear stream flowing through it. I imagine myself bathing in the pristine water, and I think of all wastes leaving me and returning to mother earth, where they are broken down into pure elemental components by the soil microorganisms.

HERBAL REMEDIES FOR YOUR LIVER

In scientific terms, herbs contain several kinds of substances that protect and fortify the liver. These fall into five classes:

1. Antioxidants, which protect cells and tissues in the liver
2. Membrane-stabilizing compounds, which protect liver-cell integrity
3. Choleretics, which promote bile and help detoxify the liver
4. Substances that prevent depletion of certain vital sulfur compounds
5. Substances that either stimulate or reduce the activity of the liver-enzyme system

Table 5 lists some herbal sources of these five types of substances. You will note that vitamins, minerals, amino acids, and flavonoids also have these five different properties so, for comparison, I have listed them under the herbs. Although many of these vitamins, minerals, and amino acids are available in synthetic supplements, I recommend obtaining them directly from herbs and foods, because plants contain these substances in forms that are more easily assimilated. Also, synthetic supplements may interfere with the uptake and utilization of other vital elements in your diet. Another advantage of natural over synthetic sources is that herbs are an excellent source of flavonoids, which are plant pigments that can strengthen blood vessels, act as antioxidants,

TABLE 5

Sources of Liver-Protecting Substances

SOURCE	ANTIOXIDANT	STABILIZING COMPOUND	CHOLERETIC	SOURCE OF SULFUR	PROMOTES ENZYMES
Plants					
Artichoke leaf	X		X		
Bilberry	X				
Cabbage	X	X		X	X
Cayenne	X				
Dandelion			X		
Garlic	X		X	X	
Ginkgo	X				
Lemon balm	X				
Licorice	X				
Milk thistle	X	X			X
Mugwort			X		
Onion				X	
Rosemary	X				
Schisandra	X				X
Skullcap	X				
Turmeric	X				
Vitamins					
A	X				
C	X				
E	X				
Minerals					
Selenium	X				
Zinc	X				X
Amino acids					
Cysteine	X			X	
Glutathione	X				
Methionine	X			X	
Flavonoids					
Catechin	X				
Kaempferol	X				
Luteolin	X				
Quercetin	X				
Rutin	X				

and impart other beneficial effects (for instance, they accumulate under the skin and protect it from ultraviolet radiation as well as reduce inflammation in the body). And last, but not least, recent studies show that herbs have enzyme-modifying effects and provide structural elements for some enzymes.

Synthetic supplements, on the other hand, neither contain nor promote the activity of enzymes, those all-important catalysts in the process of digestion.

Table 5 is designed to give you an overview of some of the active ingredients in foods and herbs that can benefit the liver. In actual practice, many herbs are taken in combinations called *formulas*. A number of formulas I have found to be helpful for specific liver-related ailments can be found starting in Part Three. You can also design your own formulas by blending together several different herbs and experimenting with taste and effectiveness.

Remember to start out with a small dose (1 cup per day of a tea) to check for individual sensitivity before working up to a full therapeutic dose (about 3 cups of tea per day: 1 cup morning, afternoon, and evening). Or simply select a good-quality ready-made product (ask your supplement department consultant) available in natural-food stores and try a bottle. It is good to follow a supplement program for up to 3 months to give it a fair trial, though you should start seeing results within 2 weeks.

When designing programs, keep in mind that herbs are usually blended together based on their "energetics." This means that some herbs are stimulating (cleansing, cooling, or warming), some are tonifying (strengthening), and some are protective. Generally, if you are weak and run-down, add tonifying herbs to specific herbs that sound right for your condition. If you are not particularly run-down or chronically fatigued, you might try a mild cleansing program with the specific herbs. If you feel hot, or have signs or symptoms of pathogenic (related to illness or symptoms) heat, add cooling herbs (most bitter herbs and formulas are cooling); if you feel cold, and your digestion is particularly sluggish, try a warming formula, such as an Indian spice tea (ginger, cardamom, cinnamon, clove, etc.). A full discussion of formulating is beyond the scope of this book, but more information can be found in many of my other books and writings.

Here is a short list of commonly used liver herbs classified according to this energetic system:

STRONG CLEANSERS	GENTLE CLEANSERS	BUILDERS	PROTECTORS	BALANCERS
Cascara sagrada	Artichoke	Milk thistle	Schisandra	Fringe tree
Butternut bark	Burdock	Reishi	Ginger	Boldo
Dock	Dandelion root	Ligustrum lucidum	Milk thistle	Bupleurum
Black root (Leptandra)	Oregon grape root	American ginseng	Turmeric	Fennel

Another aspect herbalists consider is whether an herb has a cool, neutral, or warm energy, since this will determine the types of conditions for which it can be used. For example, if a patient has symptoms of liver "fire" (headaches, red face, anger, high blood pressure, etc.), a cooling herb would be useful while a warming one might even be harmful. On the other hand, for a person suffering from liver stagnation (headaches, belching, depression, irritability, irregular menstruation, etc.), a warming herb might be beneficial. Herbal formulas that take all of these factors into consideration are presented in the next section, where specific liver-related complaints are discussed.

Table 6 presents the major liver syndromes as they are differentiated and diagnosed in TCM. I've also included modern Western correlations for these syndromes, plus a short list of herbs

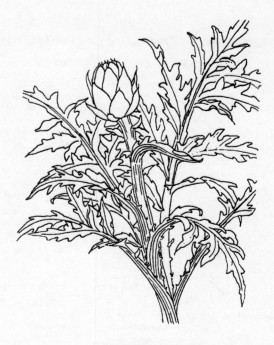

Artichoke

Cynara scolymus

commonly used for them. TCM theory is especially useful because it is so highly articulated, having been refined and tested for thousands of years. The liver "yin" refers to the actual enzymes, bile, proteins, and other substances the organ produces. When the liver is overstimulated by the need to metabolize drugs, environmental toxins, and alcohol, and to process a constant barrage of fats, its ability to produce these vital substances is reduced, creating a state of "liver yin deficiency." The liver yang refers to the actual processes of the liver, not the results of these processes, which are yin substances.

In Tables 7 and 8 (see Part Three) other herbs that may be used

TABLE 6

Liver Syndromes in Traditional Chinese Medicine

SYNDROME	SIGNS & SYMPTOMS	WESTERN CORRELATION
Stagnant liver qi	Depression, anger, frustration, irritability, temple headaches, lumps in the neck and breast, poor fat digestion, irregular menses	Congested liver, insufficient blood, reduced ability to make enzymes and other vital substances
Deficient liver yin	Dizziness, eye dryness, flushed face, irritability, ringing in the ears, warm palms and soles	Reduced enzyme and protein production, low vital energy in the liver, often accompanied by adrenal weakness
Rising liver yang	Temple headaches, dizziness, low roar in the ears, dry mouth and throat, insomnia, irritability	Headache, vertigo, tinnitis, insomnia
Blazing liver fire/ rising liver fire	Hypertension, migraine headache, dizziness, low roar in the ears, red face and eyes, insomnia, violent anger, bitter taste in the mouth	Acute conjunctivitis, heart disease, liver too metabolically active with increased heat, hepatitis, cirrhosis
Liver blood deficiency	Weak tendons and ligaments, poor digestion, irregularity or cessation of menstrual flow	Anemia, blood deficiency
Liver wind	Rigid body, ligaments, tendons, vertigo, dizziness, pain, convulsions, spasms, tremors	Hepatitis, jaundice, inflammation of the gall bladder, bile blockage

for liver and gallbladder disorders are listed with their actions as interpreted by both Chinese and traditional Western herbalism. Note that there are only a few herbs that specifically target the gallbladder, whereas there are many herbs that also target the liver. However, the double-action herbs for the liver and gallbladder together are especially stimulating to the bile and the health of the gallbladder. I realize that many lay readers will not be able to use this information to design their own herbal formulas, but I have included these tables for natural-health practitioners and students of herbalism. If you have little experience formulating or using herbs for healing, start with one or two herbs, especially mild herbs like dandelion or burdock. The majority of herbs in

Therapy	Herbs
Regulate the liver qi, harmonize the liver, choleretics to increase bile flow	Dry, fragrant herbs: burdock, cyperus, dandelion, boldo, bupleurum, fringe tree bark
Tonify the yin, cool false heat	Use sweet, moist, slightly bitter, cool herbs: rehmannia, lycii berries, tribulus, peony, American ginseng, ligustrum
Sedate the yang	Chrysanthemum flower, heal-all, skullcap herb, Chinese baical skullcap root, white peony root, epimedium leaf (yin-yang huo)
Cool liver fire	Use cool, bitter herbs: Gentian, chrysanthemum, skullcap
Tonify blood	Use neutral, blood-tonifying herbs: Lycii berries, rehmannia, dong quai, fo-ti (he shou wu), mulberry fruit (sang shen), longan fruit
Pacify liver wind, circulate blood and energy in and around the liver	Gastrodia, honey mushroom, valerian, skullcap

the following charts are mild enough in moderate doses to be used without any problem. Here are some general guidelines to remember when using the herbs.

GUIDELINES FOR HERB USE

- Start with one herb, like dandelion tea, or make a simple formula with two or three herbs at most.
- Start with a low dose and work your way up to a full therapeutic dose after a week or so if you do not experience any unpleasant side effects.

- The most common side effects of herbs to watch out for include:
  - upset stomach, gastrointestinal upset with loose stools
  - allergies with a skin rash (rarely)
  - headache
- For flowers, leaves, and other light parts of a plant, make an infusion. This is done by bringing water to a boil, taking it off the heat, adding the herbs, and then covering the pot and letting the mixture steep for 10–20 minutes. For heavier herb parts, such as the roots, bark, or seeds, a decoction is preferable. To make a decoction, simmer the herbs for 20–60 minutes.
- To judge how much herb to add to a measured amount of water, use the general formula of 1:10 (grams herb: milliliters water or ounces herb: ounces water) for decoctions and 1:20 for infusions. The ratio of herbs to water, as well as the length of time for infusing or decocting, can be varied according to need and taste. The longer an herb steeps, the stronger the tea.
- Finally, it is best to prepare herbal teas in a stainless-steel, glass, ceramic, or clay pot. Strictly avoid Teflon-coated pans and aluminum. Herbalists agree that the latter may act as a source of potentially toxic substances or affect the tea's energetic properties.
- The average therapeutic dose for most herbs is:
  - For tea, use about 4–9 grams per day of each herb in a blend or by itself. For roots, seeds, and barks (heavier materials), simmer gently for 30 minutes and then steep for 15 minutes. Strain and drink 1 cup in the morning and 1 cup in the evening. For flowers and leaves, make an infusion by steeping the herb or herb blend in freshly boiled

water for up to 30 minutes. Drink 1 cup morning and evening, before meals, to help reduce stomach upset and promote good digestion.

* For tinctures: 2–5 milliliters (35 drops = 1 milliliter or ml), 3–5 times daily in a little tea, water, or diluted juice.
* For powdered extracts or standardized extracts in capsules or tablets, follow the manufacturer's instructions on the label.

- Take the herbs consistently every day. The first "course" or period of use should be about 2 weeks for most strong herbal formulas. For tonics like ginseng and ginger, use for 1–3 months, and check back with your herbalist, or reevaluate your progress to see if you are still benefiting from the formula. If you feel no changes or benefits after 2 weeks, discontinue the formula and try another.

- If you feel some side effects, such as upset stomach, try reducing the quantity of the formula by half and continue. Often, mild side effects can mean that the herbs are working. This is known as a "healing crisis." The unpleasant symptoms should clear up after a week to 10 days. If not, you might be allergic to the herbs, or they might be the wrong ones for your present condition or constitution.

- Always consult a qualified health-care practitioner for a complete diagnosis and treatment plan, including herbal formula if you consistently experience problems with herbs. A traditional Chinese herbalist or well-trained Western herbalist can determine the best formula for you based on tongue and pulse diagnosis, along with their past experience.

three

Programs for Specific Complaints

In this part, I will give complete instructions for recognizing and remedying a variety of liver-related disorders and complaints. Tables 7 and 8 list many herbs that benefit the liver and gallbladder, and indicate their specific functions. I have experimented with these herbal formulas and natural therapies for over 30 years, and have found them to be highly effective for a great number of people, including myself. It is important to understand that herbs alone may not counteract the negative consequences of continuing bad habits. To achieve a state of optimum health, you must combine herbal treatment with proper diet, various other natural therapies, and a lifestyle that has a time and place for relaxation. Again, if your liver-related condition is serious, or if your symptoms are confusing and you are not sure which of the following programs applies to you, I recommend that you seek the help of a qualified health practitioner to explain any pathological condition in your body. If you have a serious liver condition like cirrhosis, you will want to know the details so you can plan your natural program with the help of an herbalist or qualified health-care practitioner. The team approach or "integrated medicine" affords many more choices today. Why not get someone on your team who is highly trained in disease, and one or more who are trained in health?

TABLE 7
Herbs for the Liver and Gallbladder

Common Name	Latin Name	Energy	Action
Anise seed	*Pimpinella anisum* (L.)	Warm	Mild liver protector, circulates qi
Artichoke leaf	*Cynara scolymus* (L.)	Cool	Improves appetite, reduces digestive pain, promotes bile
Baical skullcap	*Scutellaria baicalensis* Georgi.	Cold, bitter	Sedates liver yang, fire; red eyes, irritability
Barberry	*Berberis vulgaris* (L.)	Cool	Cools liver fire, hepatitis
Black root, Culver's root	*Veronicastrum virginica*, (L.), (Farw.)	Cool	Stimulates liver qi stagnation, especially with constipation
Blessed thistle	*Cnicus benedictus*, Gaert.	Warm	Stimulates liver qi stagnation with painful or difficult digestion
Boldo	*Peumus boldo* (Mol.)	Warm	Stimulates liver qi stagnation, gallstones, dyspepsia
Bupleurum (Chai hu)	*Bupleurum chinense* (D.C.), *B*. spp.	Cool	Regulates liver qi, irregular menstruation, mood swings, painful digestion; dizziness, headaches
Burdock	*Arctium lappa* (L.)	Cool	Relieves liver stagnation, tonifies liver yin; cleanses liver, especially for skin problems like eczema
Celandine	*Chelidonium majus* (L.)	Cool	Cools, detoxifies liver; jaundice

Common Name	Latin Name	Energy	Action
Centaury	*Centaurium erythraea* (Rafn.) *Centaurium* spp.	Cool	Cools the liver, stimulates bile, relieves dyspepsia, promotes appetite
Chaparral	*Larrea divaricata* (Sesse. & Moc. ex D.C.), (Coville)	Cool	Stimulates liver qi stagnation; antioxidant; some toxicity when used in high amounts, long term
Chicory	*Chicorium intybus* (L.)	Cool	Cools and cleanses the liver; skin problems related to liver heat (acne, boils)
Chrysanthemum flowers (Ju hua)	*Chrysanthemum morifolium* (Ramat.)	Cool	Cools liver inflammation; clears and cools eye inflammation; excessive tearing; tonifies liver yin
Dandelion root	*Taraxacum officinale* (G.H. Weber ex Wigg.)	Cool	Major liver herb for promoting appetite and good digestion; cools liver; cleansing to the liver
Dong quai	*Angelica sinensis* (Oliv.), (Diels)	Warm	Improves protein metabolism in the liver in people with chronic hepatitis, cirrhosis
Elecampane	*Inula helenium* (L.)	Warm	Relieves liver qi stagnation, promotes blood and bile flow; promotes tone and peristalsis in bowels; relieves dyspepsia
Fennel	*Foeniculum vulgare*, (Mill.)	Warm	Protects liver, relieves liver qi stagnation
Fenugreek	*Trigonella foenum-graecum* (L.)	Warm	Cleanses; reduces cholesterol, lubricates bowels
Fringe tree bark	*Chionanthus virginicus* (L.)	Neutral	Relieves liver qi stagnation, specific for jaundice
Fumitory	*Fumaria officinalis* (L.)	Cool	Cleanses, helps with acne
Gentian	*Gentiana lutea* (L.), *G.* spp.	Cold	Relieves liver inflammation; good for improving appetite, promoting recovery from illness; hepatitis; anorexia
Goldenseal	*Hydrastis canadensis* (L.)	Cold	Clears liver heat, removes liver stagnation, especially with constipation or loose stools; liver congestion or heat with acne, eczema, or other skin ailments
Licorice	*Glycyrrhiza glabra*, *G.* spp.	Warm	Protects the liver, anti-inflammatory effect in hepatitis
Milk thistle	*Silybum marianum* (L.), (Gaert.)	Neutral	Protects the liver, antioxidant, promotes regeneration, mild bile stimulant, liver qi stagnation
Mint, field	*Mentha arvensis* (L.)	Cool	Relieves liver qi stagnation; relieves intestinal gas
Mugwort	*Artemisia vulgaris* (L.)	Cool	Reduces heat in liver, reduces liver qi stagnation

Common Name	Latin Name	Energy	Action
Mulberry, white leaf (Sang ye)	*Morus alba* (L.)	Cold	Clears liver heat; red itchy eyes; can be used to clear liver yin deficient heat
Oregon grape root	*Mahonia aquifolium* (Nutt.)	Cold	Reduces inflammation, dampness in lower bowel, and liver; hepatitis, jaundice
Poplar bark, cottonwood bark	*Populus alba* (L.), *P. tremuloides* (Michx.), *P.* spp.	Cool (tea); warm (tincture)	Reduces inflammation, relieves qi stagnation
Skullcap	*Scutellaria lateriflora* (L.)	Cool	Reduces abdominal pain, liver protective effect
Shiitake	*Lentinus edodes*	Neutral	Acts as immunomodulation, antiviral
Wild indigo root	*Baptisia tinctoria* (R. Br.)	Cold	Antiviral, useful for acute cases of hepatitis
Wormwood	*Artemisia absinthium* (L.)	Cool	Regulates liver, promotes digestion; use infusion daily before meals for digestive pain
Yarrow	*Achillea millefolium* (L.)	Neutral	Cools fire, circulates qi; anti-inflammatory, decongesting, diaphoretic
Yellow dock	*Rumex crispus* (L.)	Cool	Relieves damp and heat in the liver and bowel; promotes elimination, regulates bowels

TABLE 8

Herbs for the Gallbladder

Common Name	Latin Name	Energy	Action
Alfalfa	*Medicago sativa* (L.)	Cool	Nutritive tonic
Artichoke leaf	*Cynara scolymus* (L.)	Cool	Promotes bile flow, enhances fat digestion, relieves digestive pain
Boldo	*Peumus boldo* (Mol.)	Warm	Moves the bile; used for gallstones
Celandine, greater	*Chelidonium majus* (L.)	Cool	Antispasmodic; relaxes bile ducts, reduces inflammation for gallbladder pain
Fumitory	*Fumaria officinalis* (L.)	Cool	Moves bile, antispasmodic for gallbladder, bile ducts for reducing pain, colic of gallbladder, gallstones
Milk thistle	*Silybum marianum* (L.), Gaert.	Neutral	Promotes bile; gallbladder pain, especially with liver or spleen inflammation
Mugwort	*Artemisia vulgaris* (L.)	Warm	Moves bile, relieves abdominal pain from cold

PROGRAMS FOR SPECIFIC COMPLAINTS

Common Name	Latin Name	Energy	Action
Prickly ash bark	*Zanthoxylum americanum* (Mill.), *Z. bungeanum* (Maxim.)	Warm	Helps relieve gallbladder pain
Spindle tree	*Euonymus atropurpureus* (Jacq.)	Warm	Moves bile, used for painful digestion and skin problems due to stagnant bile
Turmeric	*Curcuma longa* (L.)	Warm	Promotes bile, reduces gallbladder inflammation, use in formulas for gallstones
Wormwood	*Artemisia absinthium* (L.)	Cool	Moves bile, relieves painful digestion when taken as a tea

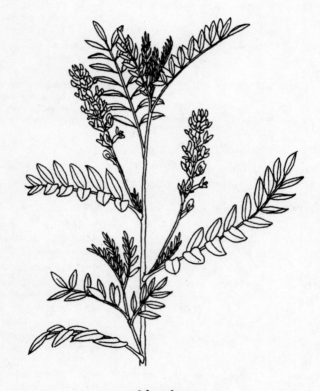

Licorice

Glycyrrhiza glabra

POOR OR PAINFUL DIGESTION (DYSPEPSIA)

Diagnostic symptoms: Soreness in the liver area under moderate fingertip pressure; painful digestion; gas pains; constipation (less than one bowel movement per day); feeling of fullness in stomach and intestines; loss of appetite; PMS; depression.

Dietary recommendations: Rest the digestive tract and liver by allowing at least 12 hours between the evening and morning meals. After 7:00 P.M., eat only small portions of fruit or drink herb tea. Exercise or do some physical work in the morning before eating breakfast. A moderate walk after a large meal will help stimulate the digestive juices. Do not overeat. Try skipping a meal (lunch), and eat light, easily digested foods such as steamed vegetables and raw salad greens (make some of these bitter). Eat semisweet fruits such as apples and pears in moderation. Add olive oil to food in teaspoonfuls and go easy on cooked or refined oils.

Do the liver flush (see page 28 for instructions) for 1 week on, 2 days off, and 1 week on. This cycle can be repeated for 1 month but not more than 2 months. Enemas are of some benefit when there is a history of heavy, refined foods in the diet.

Herbal recommendations: Take herbs that decongest the liver, increase blood flow, and have an opening, slightly warming action. I recommend the following basic formula for a decongestant tea.

Remember, this is a strong medicinal blend, and as with all such formulas, it is best to start with small doses, perhaps only several tablespoons per dose at first. Then work up to the full recommended dose after a few days, being sure to check for individual sensitivities and reactions as you go. Note that if your condition is mild, this tea is not for you; drink Polari-Tea or Puri-Tea instead (again, see the section on liver flushes, page 28). Both of these are milder, taste better, and can be taken several times a day or as desired. Simple teas or tinctures added to tea also can be useful to start. I recommend dandelion, burdock, fringe tree bark, boldo, and bitter herbs like gentian and angelica.

LIVER DECONGESTANT TEA

Dandelion root (1 part)
Fennel (½ part)
Milk thistle extract (1 capsule added to the tea or 2-3 droppers of tincture)

Burdock root (½ part or add 1-2 dropperfuls of tincture to 1 cup of tea)
Ginger (½ part)

Mix 1 ounce of whole herbs with 5 pints of water. Simmer (decoct) for 20 minutes, remove from heat, and let stand for 10 minutes before bottling or drinking. Drink ¼–½ cup of warm tea two or three times per day. For convenience, make 1 quart of tea at a time (keeping relative proportions of herbs the same), and store it in the refrigerator. Always warm up the tea before drinking it. This formula can be mixed together in powdered form and encapsulated. Take 2 capsules three times per day.

Other natural therapies: Massage the liver area by lying flat on your back and pressing your fingertips up under the right side of your rib cage. Use increasingly deep, circular motions, until all soreness or tightness is relieved. (If soreness persists for more than a week, or if there is a pronounced tenderness in the area, it may be wise to seek the aid of a skilled natural-health practitioner.)

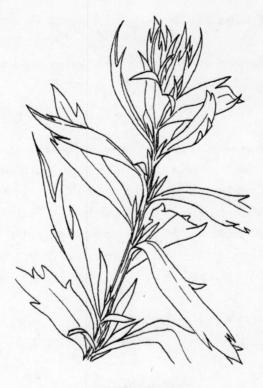

Mugwort

Artemisia vulgaris

Too much sitting and too little physical activity can block up the intestinal and liver area. Sitting and staring at a computer monitor all day is especially nefarious. Two of my greatest allies in balancing my own life in this regard are walking, stretching (such as yoga), and meditation. It is also good to massage this area often and to eat lightly until this condition improves.

POOR FAT DIGESTION

Diagnostic symptoms: Feeling of nausea or soreness in gut after fatty meals; burping with an oily taste in the mouth or throat; avoidance of or revulsion to fatty foods.

Dietary recommendations: Rest the digestive tract and take liver flushes, as explained above. One of the best and most obvious remedies is to avoid foods cooked or fried in oil. Keep diet mostly fresh—about 30 percent raw fruits and vegetables and 70 percent steamed vegetables, whole grains, and either aduki or mung beans. Try using some white organic basmati rice instead of brown rice—it's easier to digest.

Herbal recommendations: Take herbs to increase bile flow, especially the following milk thistle/artichoke combination.

PRO-BILE TEA

Milk thistle seed extract (1 part–1 dropperful or 1 tablet of the extract per cup)	Mugwort or wormwood leaf (¼ part)
	Yellow dock root powder (½ part)
Artichoke leaves (1 part)	Peppermint leaf (½ part)
Dandelion root (1 part)	Stevia herb (optional) to taste

Warm the tea to room temperature and drink ¼ to ½ cup of the tea before meals, especially fatty meals.

NOTE: It is best to buy yellow dock as whole as possible, and powder it yourself in a coffee grinder or blender. If you find the mugwort or wormwood too bitter, try substituting boldo leaf (if you can find it at a local herb show or on the Internet), or just skip it altogether. The artichoke leaf with yellow dock and peppermint will work well in most cases. You can add a little ginger and orange peel as a flavoring ingredient, or if you feel cold, as in the winter. Sweeten with stevia herb, if desired.

If nausea after fatty meals persists, it might be an indication of a deep-seated liver imbalance, in which case I recommend seeking the help of a skilled natural health practitioner.

IRRITABLE BOWEL SYNDROME

Diagnostic symptoms: Burning, cramping, or uncomfortable feelings in the bowels; alternating diarrhea and constipation; frequent gas and rumbling sounds in the intestines. These symptoms are usually worse after stress or when tired. There may be periods that are symptom-free, followed by stretches of pronounced symptoms. Bowel diseases or imbalances are extremely difficult to diagnose. Pains can move from one area of the abdomen to another. Other possible ailments showing similar symptoms include appendicitis, diverticulitis, microflora imbalance resulting from antibiotics or other chemical factors, gallstones, and even cancer. While cancer is the least likely, nonetheless, it is wise to consult a qualified health practitioner if symptoms continue for more than a week or ten days.

Dietary recommendations: Feed the beneficial flora in your intestines with foods containing ample soluble and insoluble fiber. Such foods include lightly cooked apples and other fruits, steamed vegetables, and grains that are easy to digest and are usually non-allergenic (i.e., millet, buckwheat, corn, and especially rice). Half-refined white rice is easier to digest than brown rice. Take a good probiotics supplement with a variety of beneficial organisms, such as *Lactobacillus acidophilus*, *L. rhamnosus*, *L. bulgaricus*, *Bifidobacterium bifidum*, or *Streptococcus faecium*. Make your own rejuvelac, yogurt, or sauerkraut.

Do not overeat or eat complex combinations—keep things simple. Sometimes several smaller meals during the day are easier to handle than one or two big ones. Also, eat most foods lightly to well cooked, and avoid common allergenic foods such as wheat, dairy products (especially pasteurized dairy), and eggs.

Herbal recommendations: I have had excellent results using the high-mucilage "Soothing Herbal Brew" below. Carry a quart jar with you and sip it throughout the day. Drink up to 1 quart a day (4 cups).

SOOTHING HERBAL BREW

Flaxseed (1 part)   Fenugreek (1 part)

Marshmallow root (1 part)   Caraway seed (or fennel)

Licorice root (¼ part)   (¼ part)

Simmer the ingredients in water for 40 minutes, then remove from heat and allow to steep for 15 minutes. Strain the tea and store it in the refrigerator in quart jars or other suitable containers. The tea can be used for up to 5 days, if kept cool. Drink the tea as often as possible. I carry my tea with me wherever I go, sipping it or drinking a cup every hour or two.

NOTE: If you experience cramping, add 1 part of wild yam root. Between doses of this tea, you can drink as much German chamomile tea, with or without peppermint, as you desire. I suggest up to 2 or 3 cups a day.

Other Recommendations: Be sure to follow the programs for promoting beneficial microflora recommended above. It is essential to maintain healthy microflora in any kind of bowel ailment. Research is increasingly identifying disordered microflora as a cause or contributing factor in irritable bowel syndrome and related bowel imbalances.

GAS (FLATULENCE)

Diagnostic symptoms: A bloated feeling accompanied by various pains in the abdomen or side; frequent passing of gas. Gas pains usually come and go and are not exercise related. In fact they may be relieved by movement. Applying pressure with the fingers to different abdominal areas will usually aggravate the pains. Note that gas pains can radiate into the lower chest cavity, mimicking a heart attack. If these symptoms persist or intensify, or seem to be related to activity, consult a physician.

Dietary recommendations: Keep food combinations simple. Sugars mixed with protein foods will often lead to gas. Soak legumes for one or two days before cooking. Pour off the soak water a few times and refill with fresh water. Be sure to cook beans for at least 1 hour. Note that some people cannot tolerate certain legumes, such as garbanzos or lentils. If so, then these will consistently pro-

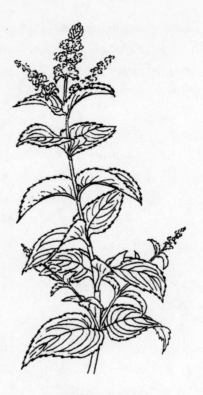

Peppermint

Mentha piperita officinalis

duce gas. Also, avoid allergenic foods, especially pasteurized milk products. Gas is a common symptom of lactose intolerance. Try taking a good *Lactobacillus acidophilus* supplement after eating dairy; substitute yogurt for milk.

Herbal recommendations: Carry a small vial of peppermint oil with you at all times. Whenever you need to, place 2 or 3 drops of this oil in a cup of hot peppermint tea or hot water, stir well, and drink. Peppermint tea is also helpful, but not as strong as the oil.

The following blend of traditional carminative, or gas-relieving, herbs is also helpful as a tea.

PASS ON GAS TEA

Peppermint (1 part)   Fennel (½ part)
Cardamom (¼ part)   Lemon peel (¼ part)
Licorice (¼ part)   Ginger (½ part)
Gentian (⅛ part)   Peppermint oil (optional)

Simmer the herbs for 20 minutes, then let the blend steep for 10 minutes, and drink as needed. Two drops of peppermint oil per cup of tea can be added for a stronger effect.

THREE-SEED TEA

Caraway seed   Cumin seed
Fennel seed   Licorice or orange peel (optional)

Steep equal amounts of the three seeds in freshly boiled water for 30 minutes, strain, and drink 1 cup after meals. You can add a little licorice or orange peel for sweetness. This is my standard formula for relieving and preventing gas. Tried and true.

Other recommendations: Beneficial bacteria should be taken consistently. Take at least 10 billion organisms per day if symptoms are severe, or 3–6 million if less severe. Some yoga postures are especially effective for relieving gas. Lie on the floor face down; put your arms under your head and your rear end up in the air. Also, try massaging the abdominal area in circular, clockwise motions.

Or, take an enema, one of the quickest remedies for gas known. The vacuum created as the enema water is expelled can literally suck out any gas caught in the bowels.

SKIN DISORDERS (ACNE, PSORIASIS)

Diagnostic symptoms: Acne or psoriasis. Skin is irritated, red, oily, itchy, and inflamed. Bowel movements may have a strong, unpleasant odor.

Dietary recommendations: Although mainstream dermatologists often do not consider diet to play a role in acne, I can assure you that it does. I suffered from acne for many years when I was younger, and I learned by trial, error, and education what did and did not work. Since then, I have used natural remedies with many people to help alleviate this problem. I have found that, as far as food goes, a diet that is 70–80 percent whole, natural, unprocessed foods is recommended. Focus on steamed and raw vegetables, whole grains, legumes, and fish or chicken (if desired). Strictly avoid processed foods with a high oil content, such as candy bars, chips, ice cream, and pizza. Consume only moderate amounts of dairy products: Eat only small amounts of cheese, use olive oil instead of butter, and avoid pasteurized cow's milk. If you do nothing else but follow this diet, I can almost guarantee results within two weeks to a month or so.

Herbal recommendations: Take cool and cleansing herbs. I like dandelion, burdock root, and burdock seed as liver/skin cleansers. Oregon grape root is a classic for skin conditions in general. Milk thistle seed extract is the most remarkable herb for psoriasis. One doctor I know who has used this extract in treating psoriasis has found that at least 50 percent of his clients improve both clinically and subjectively. Used widely in Europe, milk thistle has proved to be highly effective in protecting the liver from environmental toxins and excess free radicals. Milk thistle also works inside the liver cells to increase the production of proteins and enzymes, thus helping damaged tissues to rebuild themselves. It is a most amazing herb, and I highly recommend it. I also recommend the following tea as a general skin cleanser.

SKIN-CLEANSER TEA

Burdock root (1 part)   Licorice (¼ part)
Oregon grape root (1 part)   Fennel seed for flavor (optional)
Burdock seed (½ part)   Vitex fruit (optional)
Dandelion root (½ part)

Simmer the herbs for 20 minutes, let the blend steep for 10 minutes, and drink 1 cup morning and evening.

NOTE: I've had good clinical success with Vitex, a hormone-regulating herb that is popular in Germany for easing teenage acne. Add one dropperful of Vitex tincture per cup of tea.

Other natural therapies: Apply hot and cold hydrotherapy to affected parts. First use hot compresses, or simply splash the face repeatedly with hot water until a good flush occurs. Then repeat the process with cold water, but only with about half the number of splashes. Hydrotherapy brings fresh blood to the affected skin, stimulating a general increase of deep circulation in the area. Ideally, you should repeat this procedure several times a day. However, if that is not possible, do it at least first thing in the morning and just before retiring at night.

Hydrotherapy will also remove excess oil and dirt particles from the skin, making the use of commercial soaps unnecessary. Soap disrupts the natural protective coating of fatty acids and microflora on the skin, thus inviting pathogenic bacteria to set up camp. I have not used soap on my skin for over 15 years (except on my hands to remove grease and stubborn dirt). In that time, hydrotherapy has made my skin healthier and clearer than ever. I have also seen many other cases in which these two factors—improved circulation and proper cleansing—have eliminated chronic acne.

EMOTIONAL IMBALANCES

Diagnostic symptoms: Excessive or lingering anger, sadness, or depression. (I recommend consulting a qualified psychologist or psychiatrist, as well as a natural health-care practitioner if symptoms are persistent or more than mild, or if you have any thoughts of suicide. Then you can start on the appropriate natural program).

Dietary recommendations: Keep the liver open and clear by using liver flushes, walking and deep breathing, and the dietary recommendations outlined in Part Two. Overeating, common in excessive emotional states, only compounds the problem by further overloading the liver. The remedy is to eat lightly and to eat more fresh fruits and vegetables.

Herbal recommendations: I recommend the herbal tea listed below. St. John's wort is the major herb for mild to moderate depression. I recommend up to 3 dropperfuls of a high-quality tincture (should be dark ruby red) or up to 3 capsules of a standardized extract. Follow the manufacturer's instructions.

EMOTION-ALLY TEA

Dandelion root (1 part)

Milk thistle seed tincture
  (1 dropperful)

Lavender or rosemary herb
  (½ part)

Eleuthero (Siberian ginseng)
  (1 part)

Ginger (½ part)

Lavender (½ part)

St. John's wort (add 1–2
  dropperfuls per cup of
  tea, or take 2–3 capsules
  of a standardized extract
  separately daily)

NOTE: Sweeten with stevia herb or a little licorice. Avoid concentrated sweeteners like honey, because they can aggravate emotional swings.

Other natural therapies: Try to release "stuck" emotions in constructive ways, such as through heavy exercise or physical work. Crying and laughing, as long as they are not excessive, are helpful. Aromatherapy (the use of herbal scents) is also valuable in balancing emotional states. Try smelling lavender oil every so often during the day to brighten your spirits. I often carry a fresh, flowering top of lavender in my pocket to sniff whenever I feel the need. Bach flower remedies (a well-known aromatherapy method) work particularly well with emotional states. I recommend seeking out a Bach flower practitioner or qualified psychologist or marriage and family counselor when dealing with long-term emotional imbalances.

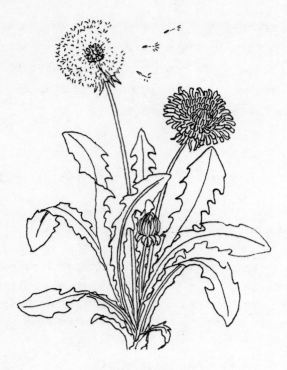

Dandelion

Taraxacum officinale

DRUG ADDICTIONS

Diagnostic symptoms: Even after an addict stops using drugs, usually some of the addictive substances remain circulating in the body for a while. This perpetuates cravings, which make kicking the habit a challenge. Both nicotine and THC (the active principle in marijuana), for instance, remain in the body long after a person quits smoking. The thing to do, then, is to eliminate all traces of old drugs from the body, a process that often takes a few weeks or even months of cleansing.

Dietary recommendations: The liver flush is ideal for removing drug-related toxins from the body. Add to this fasting with fresh vegetables and fruit juices as a means to quickly eliminate addictive substances. Fast for 3–5 days at a time, eating mostly steamed and raw vegetables afterward. See Table 4 on fasting (page 33). For extra cleansing, eat only fruits for 3–5 days before and after fasts. Some sweating and lots of fresh water and oxygen (deep breathing and vigorous exercise) will also help with the process of elimination.

GOLDENSEAL TO PASS DRUG TESTS?

A word about goldenseal: I have been asked about using this to pass drug-detection tests so many times that I've lost count. Using goldenseal in this manner has become something of a fad, and thousands of bottles of the herb are apparently being sold in health food stores all over the country for this purpose. However, according to the research that Steven Foster (1989) did on the subject, there is no clinical or laboratory basis for this use. My own theory on the matter is that beyond any placebo effect goldenseal might have (I have had people tell me emphatically that it worked for them), the herb has an overall cleansing effect on the liver, thus enhancing the body's eliminative process. If this is so, the tea and other recommendations in this section would certainly be more effective than pure goldenseal.

Do not take goldenseal during pregnancy or breast feeding.

A basic program for fast drug elimination would include bile activators (such as yellow dock, Oregon grape, and artichoke leaf), blood purifiers (such as red clover compound: red clover, burdock, dandelion, sarsaparilla), and a sauna 2–3 times in a week, using Tea-Totaler Tea during the sweat.

NOTE: If you are very weak, fatigued, and run-down, do not fast on juices but use the kitcheree fast: Eat several bowls of cooked rice with aduki or mung beans in a soupy consistency.

Herbal recommendations: Here's my formula for eliminating addictions.

"TEA-TOTALER" TEA

Dandelion root (1 part)
Wild oats (1 part–1 dropperful
  of the tincture per cup of tea)
Milk thistle tincture or extract
  (1 part–about 1 dropperful of
  tincture or 1 tablet per cup)

Passion flower (½ part)
Lobelia* (10-15 drops
  of a tincture if available)
Gotu kola (½ part–fresh
  tincture)
Ginger (¼ part)

Drink ⅛ to ½ cup of this decoction three to five times daily. Individual tinctures of the above herbs can be mixed in the proportions given to make an antiaddiction formula, if desired. Commercial herbal antiaddiction formulas are also available in natural-food stores. Decoct together in the usual way.

NOTE: The active ingredients of milk thistle, collectively called *silymarin,* are not particularly water soluble. It is best to add a tincture or powdered extract of milk thistle to the finished tea.

*Lobelia can cause nausea and vomiting in excessive doses, but it is not considered dangerous by herbalists.

Lobelia contains an alkaloid called *lobeline* that has a similar action to nicotine in the body, thereby reducing craving for tobacco in some people. I have had some good clinical success with the herb. Start with 10–15 drops and increase by 5-drop increments or until you feel a slight nausea, then reduce by 5 drops and stick to that dose.

SWEAT TEA

Yarrow tops (1 part)   Peppermint leaf (1 part)
Elder flowers (1 part)

Make 1 quart and drink 1–3 cups of the tea, warm to hot.

NOTE: Be sure to check with your health practitioner or physician before taking a sauna if you have heart disease or other imbalances that would be worsened by the high heat of a sauna. It is important to replace electrolytes (potassium and other mineral salts) lost during heavy perspiration. A good nutritional supplement with whole-food and herb extracts will work fine, or add 1 teaspoon of Dr. Bronner's Balanced Amino Bouillon to a little water and drink.

PROTECTION AGAINST ENVIRONMENTAL TOXINS

Diagnostic symptoms: Unexplained dizziness, ringing in the ears, nausea, fatigue, and "spaciness" can have a number of causes, but if they are experienced regularly, you should consider that sensitivity to chemical pollutants may be a factor. Toxic metals like lead and mercury are ubiquitous nowadays, having found their way into dental fillings and many other products. For a complete treatise on these issues, see Debra Dadd's excellent book, *Non-Toxic, Natural, and Earthwise.*

Dietary recommendations: As we've already discussed, most liver damage from environmental chemicals is thought to be due to excess free radicals. For this reason, it is good to add antioxidants and antioxidant-containing foods to the diet. I recommend vitamin E, beta-carotene, vitamin C, zinc, and selenium supplements, the latter two blended in a general nutritional supplement (not as isolated, single nutrients) during times of suspected toxic chemical stress. For regular maintenance, I suggest a program of spirulina (very high in beta-carotene), fresh greens, and liver flushes.

Herbal recommendations: The following herbal formula can be helpful. It invigorates bile flow, protects and detoxifies the liver, and stimulates phagocytosis to dispose of poisonous chemicals.

ENVIRONMENTAL SAFE TEA

Eleuthero (1 part)	Burdock (¼ part)
Fennel (1 part)	Ginger (¼ part)
Reishi (½ part)	Yellow dock root (⅛ part)
Bladderwrack (1 part)	Milk thistle tincture (add
Fenugreek (½ part)	1-2 dropperfuls)

Sweeten to taste with stevia herb or a little licorice. Decoct together in the usual way and drink ½ cup two to three times a day.

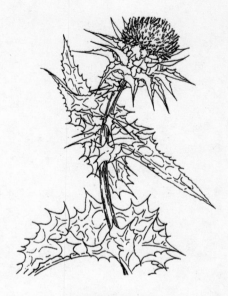

Milk Thistle

Silybum marianum

Other natural therapies: Exercise, sweating (saunas), and intestinal cleansing are useful adjuncts. One excellent intestinal cleanser is fruit pectin powder, which has been used extensively in Russia for removing environmental toxins and radiation from the body. Take 1–3 tablespoons of the powder in water or freshly squeezed fruit juice first thing in the morning and follow with 2 glasses of water or herb tea. Bentonite clay is another good bowel cleanser. Put 1 teaspoonful in a glass of water, stir, and leave the mixture in the sun for a few hours to ionize the clay's microparticles. When these particles are charged, they attract and bind toxins, thus helping to pass them from the body. One enema a day is also desirable during any cleansing.

four

Hepatitis, Cirrhosis, and Fibrosis

Note: Hepatitis is a disease that requires the attention of a qualified health practitioner or physician.

CAUSATIVE FACTORS AND BACKGROUND INFORMATION

Hepatitis is an extremely common inflammatory disease of the liver. The most frequently associated *pathogen,* or disease-causing agent, is one or more of a number of viruses, including hepatitis

A, B, C, and D. Less common viral agents of hepatitis include those associated with Epstein-Barr syndrome and yellow fever. Occasionally, herpes viruses such as varicella zoster or cytomegalovirus are implicated, as are coxsackievirus and measles virus. Bacterial hepatitis can be associated with tuberculosis, syphilis, and other systemic infections. Other pathogens, such as the protozoa that cause malaria and toxoplasmosis, and parasites that cause schistosomiasis and ascariasis, can cause liver damage but not true hepatitis.

DIAGNOSTIC SYMPTOMS

Signs and symptoms of hepatitis vary and may include extreme fatigue, headaches, facial flushing, red and inflamed gums, tenderness in the liver area, diarrhea or loose, watery stools, and yellow coating on the back of the tongue. Hypertension and migraines are also potential symptoms. Especially notable is a loss of one's normal feeling of well-being and a yellowing of the skin and whites of the eyes characteristic of jaundice.

Jaundice indicates that the liver is failing to properly break down *bilirubin,* a bile product. Bilirubin is a yellow-brown pigment that gives blood its characteristic color. If not broken down by the liver, it can accumulate in the tissues, turning the urine dark yellow or even orange. When a person is jaundiced, the whites of the eyes and even the skin are often colored yellow. Because the degraded bilirubin is no longer excreted from the bowels, the stools lose their normal brown look and turn pale to chalk white—a shock for many people.

If you experience any of these symptoms or signs, it is important that you work with a qualified primary health-care provider

TABLE 9

Classification of Viral Hepatitis and Associated Viruses

Hepatitis Type	Main Methods of Transmission	Common Outcome
Hepatitis A (HAV or infectious hepatitis)	Contamination of food, etc., with fecal matter from infected person	Often resolves completely after 4–8 weeks; usually does not become chronic
Hepatitis B (HBV or serum hepatitis)	Contaminated blood transfusions; shared needles associated with intravenous drug use	Often less favorable than type A; can be fatal in 10–15 percent of all cases in the elderly and after blood transfusions when contaminated with the virus; can become chronic in 10–15 percent of all cases
Hepatitis C (HCV)	Shared needles or contaminated blood transfusion; sexual transmission rate low, as is dental work and tattoos where blood is involved, but they are possible routes	Irregular course: patient is often asymptomatic for years; most common type of hepatitis to become chronic; different strains have been detected, some more apt to become chronic than others
Hepatitis D (HDV)	This virus is closely associated with HBV	Exists only concurrent with hepatitis B; causes extremely severe symptoms; may be an important cause of hepatitis worldwide

who can help you diagnose the ailment, define contributing factors, and develop a complete program for liver health. See table 9 for a listing of the methods of transmission and common outcomes of various forms of hepatitis.

HEPATITIS C

By far the most important cause of hepatitis is infection from one or more of the hepatitis viruses, often accompanied by an unhealthy lifestyle and other factors, such as regular or heavy alcohol or drug use. These unhealthy practices encourage a virus overgrowth that places heavy stress on the liver, making symptoms worse.

Of the hepatitis viruses, hepatitis C is emerging in many industrialized countries as a slowly developing liver infection that leads to chronic, active hepatitis. Hepatitis C is the most common blood-borne infectious disease in the United States. A study published in the October 8, 2001, issue of the *Archives of Internal Medicine* (161:2231–37) reported that the hepatitis C virus (HCV) cost the United States alone about $5.46 billion in 1997, which was similar to national health-care costs associated with asthma and arthritis. The Centers for Disease Control and Prevention (CDC) said recently that mortality associated with HCV infections could triple within 10–20 years. Hepatitis C affects at least 170,000 Americans each year.

The primary source of hepatitis C infection is needle sharing among drug addicts, and the secondary sources are blood transfusions and organ transplantation. Blood was not checked for hepatitis C before 1992. Although it is unknown how many people are infected, it is likely to be in the millions in the United States alone. Hepatitis C is especially insidious because it often takes years for infected people to demonstrate symptoms. By the time the infection is diagnosed, extensive liver damage can already have occurred.

Many people are concerned that hepatitis C may be transmitted to spouses or sexual partners. Several studies conclude that unprotected sex, even with partners who are antibody-positive to the hepatitis C virus, does not increase the risk of contracting the disease, or that such contraction is rare. The authors of one study conclude that: "While these results cannot exclude a role for the sexual transmission of HCV, they do suggest that, in this sexually active population, the sexual transmission of HCV occurs infrequently and that HCV is largely associated with intravenous drug use."

Two other studies suggest that sexual transmission of HCV is possible but probably not a major cause of infection. In the first study, researchers found only a slightly increased risk among 340 patient volunteers. In the second study, partners of HCV-positive subjects were four times more likely to be HCV-positive than those with sexual partners who were not HCV-positive. To rule out other risk factors contributing to these results, the researchers checked the identity of the RNA from virus samples of each person and found an only 12 percent higher match between the samples from sexual partners as for the random samples. HCV genetic material has been detected in saliva, semen, and vaginal discharges by one group of researchers, but not by others. There is a suggestion here that the longer sexual partners are together, the greater the risk of the disease being transmitted.

As a clinical herbalist and acupuncturist, I have specialized in this form of hepatitis and have worked with many patients suffering from it. Over the years I have observed that many people with hepatitis C can heal their livers and enjoy long, healthy lives when they utilize the total program for health described in this book.

WHAT A DOCTOR WILL DO FOR HEPATITIS

If you have symptoms associated with liver disease, it is wise to seek the help of a physician who can diagnose and evaluate your condition. The doctor will order tests that can help determine if you have hepatitis or another type of liver disease. The test most commonly requested is a liver panel, which can be ordered as part of a complete blood test (CBC) or separately. A physical examination in which the practitioner palpates the liver area to find tenderness or swelling is also useful. Here are some guidelines from the Centers for Disease Control (CDC) for who should be tested for HCV.

- People who ever injected illegal drugs, including those who injected once or a few times many years ago
- People who were treated for clotting problems with a blood product made before 1987, when more advanced methods for manufacturing the products were developed
- People who were notified that they received blood from a donor who later tested positive for hepatitis C
- People who received a blood transfusion or solid organ transplant before July 1992, when better testing of blood donors became available
- Long-term hemodialysis patients
- People who have signs or symptoms of liver disease (e.g., abnormal liver enzyme tests)
- Health-care workers after exposures (e.g., needle sticks or splashes to the eye) to HCV-positive blood on the job
- Children born to HCV-positive women

If a blood test shows that certain enzymes, called GGT, AST, and ALT, are higher than the normal range, then it is likely that the liver is under stress, either from exposure to drugs or toxic chemicals (i.e., pesticides) or from an infection—viral or otherwise. For these enzymes, Table 10 gives normal, moderately increased, and dangerously high levels.

TABLE 10

Liver Enzymes

Enzyme	Normal Range, IU/L*	Moderately Elevated, IU/L	Highly Elevated, IU/L
GGT, a biliary enzyme that is used to monitor progression of liver inflammation and disease	7-64	80-120	>120
AST (SGOT), an enzyme that increases in the blood when there is liver stress and/or damage to liver cells	10-42	80-150	150 (with severe liver damage, over 1,000 or 2,000 IU/L)
ALT (SCPT), an enzyme that increases in the blood with serious damage to cells in the liver, heart, and muscles	10-60	80-150	150 (with severe liver damage, over 1,000 or 2,000 IU/L)

Note: These values can vary, depending on the system and units of measure used.

* International units per liter

When the SGPT goes above 2,000 IU/L, the chances of developing cirrhosis are greatly increased.

In the event that your liver enzymes are higher than the normal range, and you have symptoms associated with liver stress or hepatitis, it is likely that a test will be ordered to see if you have developed antibodies to one of the hepatitis pathogens. These tests can help determine if you have been infected with HCV. Here are the most common tests. Tests that confirm the presence of antibodies in your blood that your immune system has made in response to HCV are useful, but they will not determine whether the infection is new or chronic or whether an infection is no longer present. These tests only indicate that you were exposed to the virus. Anti-HCV tests will give a positive result about

70 percent of the time after symptoms start and about 90 percent three months after symptoms begin.

Anti-HCV (detected antibodies to HCV)

Enzyme immunoassay (EIA)	Usually the first test ordered; if positive, it should be repeated
Recombinant immunoblot assay (RIBA)	Ordered to confirm a positive result on EIA

Qualitative tests such as generic polymerase chain reaction (PCR) or Amplicor HCV™ can determine the actual presence of the virus in your body by detecting HCV RNA. Quantitative tests to detect the amount of viral RNA are also available: Amplicor HCV Monitor™ and Quantiplex HCV RNA (bDNA). It's important to note that while a positive test shows that you have been infected with the virus, a negative test does not prove conclusively that you have not. The test may not always detect the virus, and you might have had an infection in the past that your body cleared. HCV can be detected as early as 1–2 weeks after you are infected.

False positives are possible with all of the HCV viral tests, so a physician should determine if you really have an infection based on these tests, in combination with liver enzyme tests, as well as taking into account your risk factors and your symptoms. If you get a positive result from your doctor but have no other signs or symptoms, your doctor should repeat the test.

Tests are also available to see how much viral RNA is in your blood. If the test is positive for a hepatitis virus and the viral load is fairly high, a liver biopsy is often recommended. This procedure can provide information about the health of your liver and what type of disease process is present.

LIVER BIOPSY: IS IT WORTH THE RISK?

According to the findings of major medical studies involving thousands of patients:

- Liver biopsies provide more useful and definitive information about the health and present condition of the liver than any other test.
- Needle biopsy with prior sonographic examination to help guide the biopsy needle is the safest procedure.

THE IMMUNE SYSTEM, FRIEND AND FOE

Some cases of hepatitis are caused by an autoimmune disorder in which the body's own immune system attacks the liver. This is especially true in people with a very strong, aggressive immune system, such as those who rarely or never get sick with a cold or flu. The body's overactive immune response to the virus may cause more damage to the liver than the virus itself. I have seen this happen in some of my patients. If this is a possibility in your case, try a regimen of ginkgo leaf extract standardized to 24 percent flavoglycosides, two–three 40-mg tablets per day, plus a few months of milk thistle and a strong antioxidant regime (see Table 3 on page 27).

Please note that it is difficult to determine if a person with hepatitis has an overactive immune system. For this reason, if you are taking immune-strengthening herbs and receive no benefit after one–two months of use, try discontinuing them. Again, with a serious disease such as hepatitis, it is important to work directly with a qualified health practitioner for a program of total health.

The liver biopsy is an important diagnostic tool for physicians in determining the severity and aggressiveness of hepatitis and other liver diseases. This procedure provides valuable information that cannot be obtained from other, less invasive tests, including ultrasound, and it promotes accuracy in the prediction of the probable outcome of the disease. A doctor may order a liver biopsy when a blood test shows that the liver enzymes are elevated, especially for longer than several weeks. Liver biopsies are also used to determine whether a specific treatment for liver disease; such as alpha-interferon therapy, has been effective or if the liver has been adversely affected by other drug therapies that are known to be toxic to the liver.

Needle biopsy of the liver is performed after a small incision is made between the ribs over the liver area. A needle is inserted to a depth of less than 2 millimeters, and a small sample of tissue is withdrawn. Afterward the patient is required to lie still for up to three hours to reduce the possibility of internal bleeding (hemorrhage). Needle liver biopsy seems to be safer than laparoscopic liver biopsy, which calls for insertion of an optical instrument into the abdomen.

As far as the patient's perspective goes, there are problems with liver biopsy. The technique is invasive and usually painful. Complications severe enough to require hospitalization can occur in approximately 4 percent of patients. In a review of over 68,000 patients recovering from liver biopsy, 96 percent experienced adverse symptoms during the first 24 hours of recovery. Hemorrhage was the most common symptom, but infections also occurred. Side effects of the biopsies included pain, tenderness, internal bleeding, pneumothorax (a collection of air or gas in the chest or pleural space that causes part or all of a lung to collapse), and, rarely, death.

Sonography used before liver biopsy significantly reduces

complications by helping to guide the biopsy needle to an exact location in the liver. In clinical studies, ultrasound was fast (required less than one minute) and definitely demonstrated the ability to reduce complications and hospitalizations after biopsy, as well as to increase the reliability of the results (definitive diagnosis made in 99.4 percent of patients).

While modern medicine maintains that liver biopsy has its benefits, few if any studies have assessed the procedure's long-term effects. Because the liver is cut and bleeds during biopsy, there will be some subsequent scarring. Biopsy is obviously traumatic and should be used only when absolutely necessary. In a holistic sense, its main benefits may lie in its shock value. If a doctor observes that your liver is 80 percent destroyed, as one patient recently reported in my clinic, then you will become surprisingly better motivated to turn your health around.

If you are considering whether or not to have a biopsy done, it is important to remember that modern medicine often does not allow for the healing potential inherent in each individual. A program for liver health includes a diet designed to alleviate liver stress or disease, plus an effective herbal formula and other dietary supplements such as antioxidants and essential fatty acids. Optimally, this program will cause the liver enzymes to return to a normal range, as well as a decreased or low viral load. The liver will get better, and a long healthy life can be anticipated. Alternately, with or without regular healthy habits in one's life, the liver may get worse and the quality and length of life be reduced.

INTERFERON THERAPY FOR CHRONIC HEPATITIS C

The major drug therapy for chronic hepatitis C involves a drug containing three kinds of alpha-interferon (Intron A). This drug slows the progression of the virus in over 40 percent of the individuals who take it by protecting the healthy cells of the liver from being infected by the hepatitis virus and retarding viral replication. Interferon is a natural immune messenger protein that is secreted by the body's immune cells in order to deal with a viral infection.

When interferon works, depending on the severity of the disease and the health of the patient, it often takes six months to a year to return liver function to normal. And post-treatment, once the enzymes and viral load are reduced, they sometimes return to the high levels present before therapy was started. Less than 20 percent of patients who respond favorably to interferon therapy have sustained responses after 6 months. Here are a few other facts you should know about interferon before deciding to start treatment:

- Side effects may include achy joints, fatigue, headaches, flu-like symptoms, and the possibility of increased anger and irritability because the emotions are often strongly affected by the drug.
- Interferon must be injected daily, or at least three times a week, for sixteen weeks. Further courses might be recommended by your doctor.
- Frequent blood work must accompany the therapy.

It may be that interferon therapy is best for getting people with very high enzymes (200–2,000) "over the hump." However interferon is used, it should always be coupled with a natural program. Two points to consider when deciding to undergo interferon therapy are the side effects impinging upon quality of life and the long-term outcome. In my experience, most people don't like interferon therapy. It's aptly named, because it interferes with the flow of life. Many of my patients have reported that not only do they ache all over and feel fatigued on the drug, but emotionally they do not feel well. In contrast, I have observed that patients with an active hepatitis C infection who have previously experienced symptoms related to the infection and who decide to follow a natural program invariably report feeling much better. Many experience heightened feelings of well-being and increased energy. Does this sound like a good trade-off for a drug that may only offer short-term decreases in viral load and liver enzymes? I remind patients that it's not about the numbers; it's how you feel through the weeks, months, and years of your life that's important.

Recently, I attended a scientific conference on complementary and alternative medicine where a doctor related a story about a prominent medical researcher from a highly prestigious university who told his audience: "Medicine is not about making a patient *feel* good; it's about curing the disease." With a mind-set like this, it's easy to understand why modern medicine is promoting interferon or interferon plus ribavirin (another antiviral drug) as the treatment of choice for hepatitis C.

Even if interferon does reduce the viral load and liver enzymes over the course of some months, it is likely that the effect does not last. I often ask my patients, "Aren't you in this for the long term?" I hope the answer is yes. I have observed patients coming into the clinic who have taken a year or so of interferon and have observed their liver enzymes fall to normal levels and the viral load drop to a low level, only to see the numbers go back up 6 months later. Science has something to say about this effect with interferon as well. In one study that randomized sixty-one consecutive patients with hepatitis C to receive either no treatment or beta-interferon (6 MU/tiw for 6 months followed by 3 MU/tiw for 6 months), after 5 years, no differences were seen in the two groups in levels of alanine aminotransferase (ALT), the number of patients who showed no trace of the virus after treatment, or the number of patients developing liver cancer. Why suffer for a year on interferon therapy for a promise of these kinds of results?

If you do decide to try interferon therapy, it is important not to drink alcohol. Several studies have shown that response rates to interferon in patients who were moderate to heavy drinkers before treatment was significantly lower, whether they quit during therapy or not, and the response rate was lowest among patients who continued to drink. Many doctors believe that interferon therapy should not be started until 6 months after stopping alcohol consumption completely.

Although many doctors maintain that interferon is the only way to reduce the amount of virus in the liver and blood and to lessen inflammation, my clinical and personal experience with a number of cases reveals quite the contrary. One case involved a forty-five-year-old man who contracted hepatitis C ten years ago from a blood infusion and was told by his doctor that the virus had destroyed 80 percent of his liver. He had been undergoing interferon therapy for eighteen months, and for six months before he came to see me, he had been taking a double dose, all to no avail. His liver enzymes did not go down, and his viral load was not reduced. The main side effect of the interferon was an out-of-control temper, which had troubled him as a young man but not in recent years. Finally, when it seemed the interferon was not working, the doctor told him to stop taking it.

About six months later, this man happened to read some of my writings on milk thistle and natural liver therapy. After consulting with me, he began a daily regimen of 600 mg of milk thistle (80 percent standardized product). Later he started to change his diet, adding more fresh fruits and vegetables. He was obviously quite encouraged when, after a few months, his liver enzymes came down to a level lower than they'd been in years. Although this was not a controlled study and thus is inconclusive, it does point out that the natural program is worth a try in every case—if not as the sole method of therapy, then at least in a supportive role to liver biopsy and interferon. With the natural program, all you have to lose are symptoms and, in some cases, the disease.

Recently other drugs have been added to interferon in an attempt to increase the long-term response rate. The most widely prescribed combination is interferon plus ribavirin (Rebetol). Up to 40 percent of patients show reduced viral loads and liver enzyme levels after 6 months of treatment. Another recent advance in the drug treatment of hepatitis C is pegylated interferon. Researchers have shown that one problem with interferon is that it doesn't last very long in the bloodstream after injection, strongly reducing its overall effectiveness. By using a chemical process called *pegylation,* interferon can stay active in the bloodstream up to a week. This treatment gives the same 6-month results as interferon plus ribavirin therapy. In Europe, pegylated interferon plus ribavirin is said to have a 6-month effective rate of just over 50 percent, and is the standard drug treatment.

Unfortunately, these treatments, especially when ribavirin is added, have many potentially dangerous side effects. And these treatments don't allow your body to heal naturally, nor do they increase your overall level of health, as is the case with a comprehensive natural program. People with a history of major depression, autoimmune diseases, uncontrollable thyroid disease, kidney transplants, or low blood counts should not receive these therapies. Anemia is the most common side effect of ribavirin, possible birth defects limit its use during pregnancy, and potential users have to use two forms of birth control as an extra measure to guard against pregnancy. Finally, nobody knows the long-term effects of antiviral therapy. The results of drug therapy are usually followed for 6 months, but at least one study showed that the 5-year benefits of beta-interferon therapy are very low. I can tell you for certain that the long-term effect of the all-natural program is the best outcome you can achieve for yourself. When you go for the highest level of health and practice health daily in your life, the long-term benefits are realized in more energy, a more positive mental and emotional outlook, and more enjoyment from life.

HEPATITIS, CIRRHOSIS, AND FIBROSIS

When hepatitis becomes chronic over a number of years, cirrhosis can result. Cirrhosis is a degenerative process of the liver that is often fatal. It involves the disruption of the normal cell structure and functions of the liver by causing the formation of scar tissue and small to large nodules. Cirrhosis most often develops as a result of chronic active hepatitis, chronic alcohol and drug abuse, or exposure to liver toxins. In the United States, cirrhosis is the third leading cause of death among people aged forty-five to sixty-five, after heart disease and cancer.

The path to changes in the liver that lead to cirrhosis is usually a long one, perhaps covering decades. Today even children are exposed to toxic chemicals, aspirin, and other liver stressors that can start the process. Cirrhosis, ironically, has a lot to do with the natural response of the body to toxins or pathogens and with the liver's ability to heal itself. When the liver is stressed, inflammation (called "pathogenic heat" in Traditional Chinese Medicine) often results. Inflammation is the body's natural response to many potentially harmful agents. However, when inflammation continues over a period of time, the body is obviously unsuccessful in eliminating the offending agents. For instance, when the liver is chronically irritated by alcohol, the body often tries to heal or protect itself by telling specialized cells, called *fibroblasts,* to produce a tough fiber known as *collagen.* This process, called *fibrosis,* is common throughout the body as a response to chronic irritation or injury and subsequent inflammation. The scars that form after a wound and the subsequent repair process are related to fibrosis.

Imagine the liver working constantly to process alcohol, drugs, and rich fatty foods, while at the same time attempting to keep up with its many other important functions, including the manufacturing of immune proteins, the processing of natural body steroids and other chemicals, the storing of energy in the form of glycogen, and the storing of fat-soluble vitamins. When it's trying to handle all these duties, while constantly responding to the toxic compounds with which it is bombarded, the liver becomes overheated, and inflammation occurs.

Sometimes these processes lead to abnormal fibrosis, in which fibrous tissue spreads over and replaces healthy tissue. If fibrosis continues for years, the collagen fibers begin to condense and thicken until the condition becomes so extensive that bands of fibrous tissue occur. A particular characteristic of cirrhosis is the formation of small (less than one-third of an inch) to large (two-inch) nodules that may contain blood vessels and liver cells. When nodules begin to form, the liver's natural internal structure becomes disrupted, and it loses the ability to perform its normal and vital duties. The sad fact is that this process is often irreversible and can lead to death. Unfortunately, many people remain largely free of symptoms for years, often until the process is highly advanced. Some may experience only fatigue and headaches, symptoms common to many other imbalances that don't necessarily indicate that something is wrong with the liver.

The list of liver stressors associated with cirrhosis is extensive, and most people choose one or more items from it daily, even if they are not aware of it. Alcohol abuse tops the list and is implicated in most cases of cirrhosis. It is important to note here that if you have a history of symptoms associated with the liver, or if you have indulged in alcohol, drugs, poor nutrition, or other liver stressors for more than ten years, a total program for liver health is for you! Other factors in the etiology of liver disease include the frequent use of aspirin, acetaminophen, and other pain-relieving drugs, antibiotics, steroids, and exposure to toxic chemicals of any kind.

The healing of cirrhosis is difficult to predict, as it obviously depends on many factors, including a willingness to develop an excellent and consistent program for total health, a specific program for liver health as detailed in this book, and the ability to permanently eliminate any possible liver stressors, especially alcohol and drugs. The individual's constitution, innate vital energy, attitude, support group, and healthy relationships are also extremely important. With cirrhosis, it is usually impossible to eliminate the scarring and nodules, but the disease process can at least be stopped, allowing the liver to regenerate some of its vital function. My experience strongly suggests that the people who follow the most stringent program—those who walk the straight and narrow with an excellent diet and health habits—do the best; sometimes they can accomplish near miracles.

Dietary and herbal treatments for cirrhosis are virtually the same as those for hepatitis, and the patient must be correspondingly faithful to a total health program. Attention to detail is often important for optimum results.

ALCOHOL AND THE LIVER

Most doctors and herbalists alike will agree that your best plan is to completely abstain from alcohol if you have a liver disease like hepatitis C. I believe this is absolutely essential. A connection between alcohol abuse and hepatitis C infection may exist. Up to nearly 20 percent of alcoholics have antibodies to hepatitis C, which is nearly ten times the general population (1.8 percent). In other words, alcohol use might increase your susceptibility to infection with the virus. Also, hepatitis C patients who are also drinkers tend to sustain more liver damage in the process than nondrinkers. Some research seems to indicate that alcohol is actually synergistic to hepatitis C. Alcohol consumption might lead to an underlying condition that encourages viral growth and makes it more damaging. In Traditional Chinese Medicine, regular alcohol use is thought to contribute to such conditions as liver yin deficiency and liver fire. These conditions can damage your liver and lead to a whole host of symptoms such as irritability and chronic headaches.

DIETARY RECOMMENDATIONS
FOR A HEALTHY LIVER

First, remove the dietary stress factors that contribute to liver inflammation: excessive alcohol, drugs, or fried, spicy, and heavy foods such as large quantities of red meat or frequent fatty meals. These factors make it more likely that the liver will become actively infected by the hepatitis virus.

Foods and Food Supplements

A light diet built on greens, grains, and legumes is best. Don't eat too many raw foods; instead, steam them lightly The best way to get a good supply of the enzymes, vitamins, and other factors that may be destroyed during cooking is to juice vegetables. About 8 ounces of mixed vegetable juices is optimal for most people. Start with about 30–50 percent carrot juice and add some cooling, detoxifying, and mineral-rich vegetables like cucumber, celery, and parsley. Beet juice is a good blood-builder but contains oxalic acid, which can irritate the throat; add no more than 10 percent. Try the recipe for Liver-Support Juice (page 90) for starters.

"Superfoods" rich in micronutrients and high-quality proteins are essential. These include steamed nettles, spirulina or other blue-green algae, and whole almonds (soaked in water overnight if your digestion is weak). Walnuts also contain valuable proteins and omega-3 fatty acids that can help decrease inflammation in the body. Keep the eliminative channels open by drinking plenty of pure water. Avoid spicy, warming foods such as garlic, cayenne, hot peppers, and curries. If you feel like you can't live without tangy foods, use ginger as a substitute. Let food cool to almost room temperature before eating. Also avoid cooking foods in fat or oil for a while—steam or boil them instead. Although red meat can be excessively heating, according to Traditional Chinese Medicine, the liver still needs protein for regeneration, as do all the cells of the body. I recommend eliminating red meat from the diet during an acute phase of hepatitis; afterward, if desired, it can be taken in moderate amounts once or twice a week. Fish is an excellent protein source because it is easy to assimilate and is neutral or cooling to the liver. Chicken and turkey in moderate amounts can also be beneficial.

LIVER-SUPPORT JUICE

Carrot 45%	Cabbage 10%
Beet 5%	Parsley 10%
Celery 25%	Ginger 5%

NOTE: These percentages are approximate; blend the vegetable juices to taste. The ginger, which is optional, makes the juice rather spicy and is a good liver protector. You can also add a bit of apple juice for sweetness and flavor.

THE IDEAL DIET

For the liver, keep it simple. An example of what not to have for dinner would be rich casseroles with meat and oil, lots of different vegetables and chopped nuts, topped off with a sweet dessert like cake. Optimal for the liver is a simple meal of steamed vegetables and a grain like rice or millet. Even white rice can be helpful because it is easy to digest and cooling and calming for the liver. For variety, whole grains, such as millet, buckwheat, rice, quinoa, and amaranth are also beneficial. Bread is fine for some people who have little problem with wheat, but stick to whole-grain bread, freshly made and organic if possible.

HEALTHY RESTAURANT FOOD: AN OXYMORON?

Over the years I have often heard from people who travel frequently that it is difficult to maintain a healthy diet when eating in restaurants. My experience is quite the contrary. Many restaurants offer some healthy choices and flexibility in preparation and are happy to oblige their customers. Ask for vegetables with no butter or salt, perhaps steamed or stir-fried in olive oil. Fish and other main dishes can be cooked without sauces; dressing for salads can be ordered on the side and sprinkled on for flavor instead of ladled into the bowl.

Larger cities usually offer a variety of natural-food restaurants. A close friend of mine had hepatitis C for a number of years and became very sick. She had to quit her job and focus on healing her liver. She was very good at monitoring her diet and could fluster any waiter with specific instructions on how the meal should be prepared: no spices, not even pepper; very little oil; only the freshest ingredients. We made quite a pair when we were eating out together. I like some spice, but wanted fresh organic vegetables whenever possible, no meat except fish, no eggs or butter. To make up for the aggravation we caused, we tipped generously!

Eat according to the seasons. When the weather is cold, eat warmer, cooked foods. Alaskans, for example, need meat and fat in their diets, whereas South Americans need cooling fruits and vegetables. It is also important to tailor your diet to the type of work you do. Doing hard physical labor requires stronger, heavier foods than does sitting at a computer. People generally grow up eating the diet they get from their parents. Sometimes this diet is influenced by advertising such as "Milk does a body good." Milk is not good for everybody. Its benefits depend on genetic heritage, digestive capacity, and the type of work done. Sometimes people just follow their parents' diet without really examining it until they get older, start feeling aches and pains, and realize that their diet may not necessarily be right for them. The ensuing years are a time of self-discovery and figuring out one's optimum diet based on individual needs, climate, and profession. See table 11 for general guidelines.

TABLE 11

Foods to Use and Avoid for Those with Hepatitis or Cirrhosis

Foods to Use

- Steamed green vegetables
- Fresh vegetable juices
- Squashes
- Whole grains
- Legumes, including tofu, tempeh, and soups with aduki and mung beans
- Fish, organic chicken, and turkey
- Plenty of fresh water; add juice of half a lemon to 1 quart of distilled water
- Fresh fruit in season, 1-3 pieces a day, depending on season and climate

Foods and Drugs to Avoid

- Alcoholic beverages of any kind
- Consume only moderate amounts of spicy foods such as chili peppers, raw onion, and black pepper. Ginger and turmeric are preferred spices because they have protective effects on the liver.
- Pain-relieving drugs such as aspirin and products containing acetaminophen—many are toxic to the liver.
- Most pharmaceutical drugs, especially anti-inflammatories and antibiotics—check the *Physician's Desk Reference*, available in a home edition and at most libraries, if you are uncertain about the potential toxicity to the liver.

- Cannabis use should be very moderate for people with an overactive response to the virus accompanied by inflammation. Studies show that marijuana is an immune stimulant that can increase your immune system's hyperactivity.
- Fried greasy foods—they are often difficult for the liver to handle.
- Stimulants like coffee, black tea, or ephedra (ma huang) products—they increase body metabolism and act as central nervous system stimulants, increasing body heat and possibly inflammation.
- Products and foods with added refined sugar of any kind such as cakes, cookies, candy, and ice cream—Avoid foods with white sugar, honey, and maple syrup. Refined sugar suppresses the immune system, stimulates metabolism, and increases heat in the body. Depend on fresh fruit in season for natural sweets.

Nutritional Supplements to Add
- Antioxidants such as milk thistle, vitamin E (400-800 IU per day), vitamin C (1-3 grams per day), grapeseed extract (150-200 mg per day)
- Essential fatty acids—Be sure there are enough in your diet. Use 1 or 2 teaspoons of organic flaxseed oil a day on salads or steamed vegetables, or take capsules.
- B vitamins are important for liver health. Take a B-vitamin complex supplement that contains thiamine, choline, riboflavin, and niacin.

HERBS FOR THE LIVER

An effective herbal formula is often made up of several components. Each part has a specific function, or action type. An herbal formula for people with hepatitis may contain herbs with a number of different action types, depending on the person's constitution and current health.

Here are some specific formula components that have been proven effective through scientific studies and clinical experience.

Antiviral Herbs to Help Protect
Liver Cells from Viral Infection

Lemon balm tea: 2–3 cups of strong tea per day

St. John's wort: 1 teaspoon of tincture in a little water or tea two or three times daily; or 3 tablets of powdered extract per day.

Shiitake powdered extract in capsules or tablets: Take at least 2 and up to 5 grams per day. Note: A "00" size capsule contains ½ gram of powdered herb. Shiitake in combination with milk thistle is one of the most effective herbs I've used in my over 12 years of working with hepatitis patients.

Garlic, taken fresh, cooked, or in capsules: Any commercial garlic product should have some garlic smell for full antiviral effect.

Other antivirals: Consult an herbalist before taking *Baptisia* or *Lomatium* isolate. These powerful herbs are available in most natural-food stores, but they are very strong.

General Protective and Rebuilding Herbs for the Liver

Milk thistle is the major herb for hepatitis; take it as a tablet in concentrated, powdered extract form. An average therapeutic dose of the 75–80 percent standardized extract is 1 tablet three or four times daily. Also available is a 10 percent standardized extract often blended with other liver-protective and healing herbs, such as turmeric, artichoke leaf, gentian, and ginger. Of this preparation, take 1 or 2 tablets, three times daily. I prescribe up to 1 gram of milk thistle extract a day for some patients who have very high liver enzymes, say in the range of over 150, or high viral loads, over 1 million. I have never seen any appreciable side effects at this dosage, even when the herb is taken for extended periods. For more information on milk thistle, see the Appendix.

You can use schisandra in teas, taking 4–12 grams daily, depending on body weight, or as a powdered extract. Avoid alcohol tinctures of schisandra during the acute phase of hepatitis.

Other protective liver herbs: ginger, turmeric, *Eclipta alba*, fringe tree bark.

Herbs to Prevent Liver Congestion
(Bile-Moving Herbs)

These herbs include artichoke leaf, yellow dock, burdock, and dandelion root.

Herbs to Cool the Liver and Reduce Inflammation

Herbs for cooling the liver should be added to these three basic formulas in the acute stages of hepatitis, when "pathogenic heat" (active inflammation) is affecting the liver. Cooling herbs include gentian, yellow dock, Oregon grape root, centaury, coptis, and *Scutellaria baicalensis* (Chinese herbs). To determine if your liver is inflamed, consult with a licensed acupuncturist or herbalist trained in an energetic-based system of natural medicine, such as Traditional Chinese Medicine or Ayurveda.

Use cooling herbs in tea or as a powdered extract (dried tea) in capsule or tablet form. For tea, simmer 50–100 grams of cooling herbs in about 20 ounces of water for 45 minutes. Steep the herbs for 15 minutes, strain and drink 1 cup of the tea two or three times daily. The herbs will be bitter, a property associated with the cooling effect. For sweetness, add 3–7 grams of licorice, which also has an antiviral and anti-inflammatory effect.

Capsules or tablets of the dried teas (powdered extracts) of cooling herbs are available in natural-food stores and herb shops. These extracts are much more potent than dried herbs ground up and placed in capsules or tablets because they contain the active ingredients of the plants, minus the sugars and cellulose and other fibers that make up the bulk of most herbs. In other words, the extraction process concentrates the herb's activity many times.

Once the acute phase of hepatitis has passed, eliminate the

cooling liver herbs from your regimen. Keep taking the other herbs and supplements for another month or two, especially the basic supportive one. Bile-moving herbs are still appropriate in many cases.

NOTE: If hepatitis becomes chronic, I recommend working with a qualified natural health-care practitioner or holistically minded physician to design an ongoing herbal formula that contains liver-building herbs, enzyme-lowering herbs, bile movers, and appropriate dietary supplements. Such a person can order tests and provide nutritional and herbal guidance during the healing process.

COOL THE LIVER TEA

Dandelion root, raw or
  dried (not roasted), 1 part
Artichoke leaves, 1 part
Oregon grape root, ½ part

Licorice, ¼ part
Turmeric, ¼ part
Gingerroot, fresh, ⅛ part
Gentian root, ⅛ part

Simmer the herbs in a covered pot for 20 minutes. Remove from the heat and let steep, covered, for 10 minutes. Drink 1 cup morning and evening and one more, if desired. Persist as long as you experience benefits.

NOTE: This tea can be used long-term for chronic hepatitis or once an acute phase of hepatitis has passed. Dried extracts of the individual herbs or entire formulas containing many or all of the herbs in capsules or tablets are available in most health food stores and herb shops.

LIVER-SUPPORT TEA

Milk thistle, 35%

Artichoke leaf, 15%

Turmeric, 15%

Schisandra, 15%

Shiitake, 15%

Licorice, 5%

Simmer the herbs in a covered pot 20 minutes. Remove from heat and let steep, covered, for 10 minutes. Drink 1 cup morning and evening and one more if desired. Persist as long as you experience benefits.

HEPATITIS B AND C—IS THERE A CURE?

One must be careful with the word cure. *When someone is cured of pneumonia, no trace of disease is left in the body. If someone has hepatitis C and all the symptoms go away,* and an antibody test proves negative, and there are no signs of other viral activity in the body, and the liver enzymes are normal, then modern medicine might say the infected person has been cured. Yet it is likely that the hepatitis pathogen remains in the body. Millions worldwide carry the hepatitis C virus and are not aware of it. Some will go on to have symptoms, even develop serious disease, and some may remain free from symptoms into their old age. We simply don't know the percentages yet.*

One can focus on disease, or one can focus on health. If the concept of disease consumes our minds and takes a lot of attention, we are giving power to the disease. When we focus on health and its whole process, we are creating greater health instead of becoming fearful.

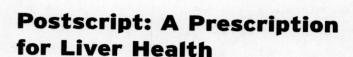

Postscript: A Prescription for Liver Health

Congratulations! If you've read this far, you've learned a lot about the liver and natural liver therapy. Here's a final summary of the most important points you should remember about regaining or maintaining liver health.

Nine Important Points for Optimum Liver Health

1. Eat a natural-foods diet of high-quality fresh food with lots of variety. Lower your fat intake. Eat less refined, cooked oils and fats. Obtain essential oils from whole nuts and seeds.

2. Rest the digestive system whenever possible. Don't eat too late at night or too early in the morning. Don't eat when not hungry, and especially never overeat.

3. Be aware of proper food combining. Sweet fruit with cooked protein is the worst combination, causing fermentation.

4. Liver flushes and drinking lemon-water keep the liver moisturized and free flowing.

5. Keep the eliminative channels open and free. Exercise to eliminate toxins via the lungs and skin. Have at least one bowel movement a day.

6. Massage the liver area at least once a day to help remove congestion.

7. Worry or anger can get stuck in the liver. Release these emotions in a constructive way.

8. Antioxidants such as vitamins E and C, beta-carotene, zinc, and selenium protect against toxins. Herbal antioxidants are superior to synthetic vitamins, though both can be used together.

9. Herbal formulas to cleanse, protect, and stimulate the liver are highly recommended. Teas for long-term use include a blend of roasted dandelion, chicory, and ginger; Puri-Tea; Polari-Tea; or any of the other teas in this book. Milk thistle is a must for rebuilding the liver when it has been compromised or weakened in any way.

When we're afraid we have a disease that can't be cured, we are likely to grope for anything—drugs, surgery, even herbs—in hope of a panacea. But disease and health are processes inside of us, not outside. By looking deeply we may come to understand our processes and help to heal ourselves.

It is always important to remember that modern medicine is limited in its ability to consider the human spirit and the vital energy that people are able to direct to their healing. Practitioners of modern medicine, as well as other kinds of practitioners, often can't foresee whether people can heal themselves or not. I feel, however, that there is no limit to what is possible with the healing process and the human spirit, so why place limits? Why close ourselves off from reaching for the health that, by making the reach, we may well attain?

APPENDIX:
MILK THISTLE

Further Information on the Liver Herb

INTRODUCTION

Medicinal herbs are still used by the majority of the population in the world today for prevention of disease and restoration of wellness. Nine hundred million Chinese people still rely on herbs for a major part of their health care. In the United States herbs have been largely supplanted by chemical drugs, but their use is becoming increasingly widespread due to the popularity of the health food movement.

This appendix will describe one medicinal herb, *Silybum marianum*, that has attracted much interest in recent years, especially in Europe, where commercial preparations are being manufactured for severe liver diseases like hepatitis and cirrhosis, as well as for liver restoration. Our modern environment is full of stressful chemicals, such as food additives and pesticides. These chemicals need to be processed by the liver so that they can be eliminated by the body. Furthermore, the liver is an important organ in the digestion of fat, which is usually overabundant in the modern diet.

It is hoped that this appendix will increase awareness and use of this herb, which grows commonly as a "weed" throughout the country.

HISTORY

Through the ages, various thistles have been thought of as part of the ancient curse of civilization and are mentioned as such in the Bible. After Adam and Eve ate the apple, God said: "Thorns also and thistles shall it bring forth to thee." They are a sign of rich land gone wrong. Bristly and prickly, they spread rapidly and cover vast fields. However, thistles can be considered a blessing as well as a curse, for since ancient times, many thistles were widely used for their curative effect on the liver and recently chemical compounds from the seed of one thistle—*Silybum marianum,* the milk thistle—have proven its ability to protect and rebuild the liver.

The ancients revered milk thistle. The Greek herbalist Dioscorides wrote that a tea of the seeds could be drunk for snake bites. Gerard, the famous English herbalist, wrote: "My opinion is that this is the best remedy that [grows], against all melancholy diseases." (*Melancholy* comes from *melanos,* meaning "black," and *chole,* meaning "bile"—an old reference to any liver- or bile-related disease.) Culpepper thought milk thistle good for removing obstructions of the liver and spleen. He recommended the infusion of the fresh root and seeds against jaundice.

The Eclectics, a school of medical herbalists of the late nineteenth and early twentieth century, used it widely for varicose veins and congestion in the pelvis, especially for menstrual difficulty and for congestion in the liver, spleen, and kidneys. They recommended five-drop doses of the tincture three times a day, until relief is obtained. The remedy acts slowly, so it must be taken persistently. Silybum was also a popular garden plant, valued for its edibility as well as its medicinal attributes.

HUMAN STUDIES

Today, there are a substantial number of scientific studies showing the effectiveness of some herbal remedies or "phytomedicines" (meaning clinically useful remedies from whole herb extracts) for relieving some medical conditions and symptoms in humans, as well as clearly demonstrating their safety.

Popular herbs such as ginkgo, saw palmetto, and St. John's wort have all been the subjects of double-blind, placebo-controlled, randomized studies—the "gold standard" of modern medical science for proving the efficacy and safety of drugs that are prescribed by physicians and paid for by government-funded health care.

Since the 1970s, milk thistle has joined their ranks and has been the subject of clinical human studies to try to demonstrate its effectiveness for extending life, improving quality of life, reducing the symptoms of hepatitis and cirrhosis, and protecting the liver against toxins in drugs and the environment. The studies have shown varying results, some revealing benefits and some not. But, at this stage, milk thistle has been studied enough to at least strongly suggest its benefits for treating some kinds of liver ailments and symptoms. Given the non-toxic nature of milk thistle preparations, further research is definitely warranted.

A few studies since 1989 involving groups of patients with chronic liver diseases have yielded good results revealing milk thistle's role in promoting enhanced liver and immune functions; an antioxidant and free-radical scavenging effect in the liver; reduced liver enzymes; and relief of symptoms such as fatigue, abdominal pressure, poor appetite, nausea, and itching. High-quality studies with large enough groups of patients to prove or disprove effectiveness have not yet been funded or performed.

PHARMACOLOGY

Milk thistle's long-standing reputation led Dr. Madaus and Company in Germany to produce an herbal preparation for liver-related diseases. This, in turn, led to an investigation of its efficacy and action by Dr. Magliulo (1973). He demonstrated stimulated regeneration in the livers of rats from whom this organ was partially removed, when he gave them an extract of silybum, called silymarin. Silymarin is the collective name by which the primary group of active chemical isomers of silybin is known. The isomers are silybin, silydianin, and silychristin, with silybin being the most frequently used in clinical applications. The mechanism of this silymarin action was not made clear until 1980, when Dr. Sonnenbichler, from Munich, showed in in vivo tests that silymarin leads to increased protein synthesis in liver cells as a result of an increased activity of ribosomal RNA via the nucleolar polymerase A.

Ribosomes are the cellular organelles where proteins are synthesized. There are three enzyme systems in most animal cells to facilitate this process:

- **Polymerase A** (for transcribing ribosomal genes from DNA to produce more ribosomes)
- **Polymerase B** (for messenger RNA that transfers the genetic information from DNA to the ribosomes where proteins are synthesized)
- **Polymerase C** (for transfer RNA, which helps connect the amino acids together in the proper sequence to form proteins and enzymes in the cell)

These enzymes and other proteins are integral to the life processes of the cell and ultimately the whole body.

Part of the silybin molecule has a steroid structure. Steroids enter the cell and stimulate the induction of new DNA and ribosomal RNA synthesis. This may be the mechanism by which silybin (a unique kind of flavonoid called a *flavanolignin*) works. Flavonoids are very common bioactive compounds, many of which are plant pigments (rutin from buckwheat is an example). Flavonoids have the basic structure:

The flavanolignans are produced in the plant by a coupling of a flavonoid and coniferyl alcohol. Coniferyl alcohol is a common phenolic compound widely used by plants as precursors to more complex molecules (the structural material lignin contains many of these units). The structure of silybin is consequently more complex:

Dr. Vogel, a leading researcher of silybum, has concluded that silybin is a representative of a new class of bioactive compounds. Flavonoids are well known to have blood vessel–toning effects, reducing fragility and permeability in them. They also have shown anti-inflammatory effects, but silymarin shows none of these properties. Instead, its action is almost entirely on the liver and kidneys. The evidence for this is that *enteral* (intestinal) absorption of silymarin is around 50 percent in humans, renal elimination (via the urine) is slight (5–7 percent), and the concentration of silymarin in the peripheral blood is slight. Silymarin is subjected to a pronounced *enterohepatic circulation* (an intestinal to liver loop). It moves from the blood plasma to the bile and is concentrated in the liver cells. This cycle is difficult to break, a reason why some toxic substances (such as alpha-amanatine, the Amanita mushroom toxin) are so destructive, and why silymarin is so effective.

Alpha-amanatine inhibits the glomerular filtration rate in the kidneys, which results in increased blood concentration of urea and other substances (waste products that can be toxic). Silymarin counteracts this, causing the plasma concentration of urea to drop. Fortunately, silybin is absorbed slowly when orally administered to various animal species, including humans, and even in large doses, no toxic effects have been noted.

The early groundwork on Silybum by Magliulo, Sonnenbichler, and others has been followed by hundreds of further studies. Representative of this research is Dr. Vogel's work with the most virulent liver toxin known, the above-mentioned alpha-amanatine from the deadly Amanita mushroom.

Some Amanitas, like A. *phalloides* (the death cup), a common U.S. species, contain two toxins. The first, phalloidine, is a virulent liver poison that destroys the outer cell membrane of the *hepatocytes* (liver cells), which can lead to death within a few hours. The second, alpha-amanatine, penetrates the cell nucleus and inhibits the polymerase-b activity, thereby preventing the synthesis of the messenger RNA, blocking ribosomal protein synthesis and leading to death after 3–5 days.

Silymarin is capable of both preventing phalloidine from reaching its receptors in the membrane (by occupying its binding sites) and transforming the outer hepatocyte membrane in such a way that alpha-amanatine is no longer capable of permeating the membrane. This breaks the enterohepatic circulation of alpha-amanatine, protecting the as yet undamaged liver cells from renewed poisoning. Vogel and coworkers showed that regeneration of alpha-amanatine–damaged rat livers is accelerated by a factor of four with silymarin, in comparison with untreated controls.

In the 1970s, Vogel conducted a remarkable study. He brought in sixty patients suffering from severe Amanita poisoning from around Europe and treated them with water extracts of 20 mg/kg of silybin a day. Because of humanitarian considerations, no controls were used. Dr. Vogel states that the "results ranged from amazing to spectacular": All of the patients treated with silybin lived. Even with modern supportive measures (using activated charcoal to absorb toxic-laden bile), the death rate is usually 30–40 percent.

One remarkable fact was that these patients were mostly treated from twenty-four to thirty-six hours after poisoning, so liver and kidney damage had already occurred. A preparation for injection based on silymarin is now undergoing clinical research by Dr. Madaus and Company for cases of Amanita poisoning in humans.

Amanita phalloides is a common mushroom of the West Coast of the United States and is increasing rapidly in numbers. It was nearly unknown five years ago, having been introduced from Europe and the Eastern United States, where it is well known.

In the fall of 1983 in the San Francisco Bay area, twenty Laotian refugees were stricken with Amanita poisoning. Several families ate a soup containing the mushrooms, which resembled ones that were considered safe in their homeland; fortunately, they all survived. Since 1981, thirty-six cases of *Amanita phalloides* poisoning have been reported in the Bay Area alone; five of the victims died. Unfortunately, silymarin therapy has been unknown in this country, but the Poison Control Center in Washington, D.C., has been experimenting with it.

Tests with silymarin have raised other therapeutic possibilities. Recent double-blind studies with cirrhotic patients proved that the survival period was prolonged and the survival rate was significantly increased by silymarin. Other studies have shown liver protection from various other drug and heavy-metal poisonings. The reference list under Notes on page 119 is comprehensive.

Silymarin also has shown a strong antioxidant effect in a number of animal and some human studies. Free radicals are highly reactive molecules with an unpaired electron. The free electron makes the molecule more unstable and it seeks strongly to share another electron from other molecules, often damaging or disrupting cells and tissues in the body in the process. Antioxidants are protective substances like vitamin C and E that can protect against the damaging effects of free radicals. Milk thistle is a potent antioxidant, and because silymarin concentrates in the liver tissues and is eliminated by the body through the bile, it delivers the antioxidant effects where it is needed most to protect the liver from damage from the free radicals generated due to exposure to noxious chemicals and viral infection.

BOTANY AND APPEARANCE

Silybum marianum is a member of the Compositae, the composite or daisy family. It is closely related to other thistles, including *Cirsium vulgare* (common thistle), *Centaurea* spp. (star thistle), and *Cynara scolymus* (artichoke). All of the thistles are edible and are known for benefiting the liver, though other than silybum, none of them are known to contain silymarin. Silybum is a stout thistle, growing from four to ten feet tall, depending on growing conditions. It has large prickly leaves marked with many undulating white zones. The flowering heads at the end of the stalks are large, bright purple, and beset with an abundance of stout spines.

ORIGIN AND DISTRIBUTION

Originally from western and central Europe, milk thistle has made itself quite at home in this country. It was once widely cultivated for its food value and has consequently escaped, now growing wild in many southern areas, including southern Europe, Africa, India, China, and South America. In California, it has been introduced and now grows widely as a weed, especially abundant from the San Francisco Bay Area south to Southern California, thanks to its great distribution system—thousands of parachuted seeds.

It prefers sunny locations, well-drained soil, and takes readily to cultivation, though because of its abundance in the wild, it hardly seems worth the trouble for personal use. Milk thistle has been cultivated in Texas for a large European company and as the demand increases in the United States, cultivation will become a necessity. It has the advantage, commercially speaking, of being very easy to start, having few predators, and providing a mature crop in less than a year.

Silybum's present growth range is from Vancouver Island to Mexico and east to the Atlantic, though it is less abundant there. It also grows in South America and Australia. In fact, much of the commercial seed production for the European market comes from Argentina.

The plants flower from March in Southern California to July or August in the Pacific Northwest. According to a two-year study by Voemel in Germany, the southern plants produce the seeds highest in silymarin. The seeds of wild plants from Turkey and Germany were analyzed—the Turkish seeds had a silymarin content "markedly higher" than that of the German plants. When wild German plants were grown in Turkey, the silymarin content was higher than normal but not as high as the wild Turkey strains in their native environment. Turkey is about the same latitude as the San Francisco Bay area, Germany about the same as Seattle.

Conditions such as rainfall, average temperature, and the genetic heritage of the plants also affect the production of silymarin by the plant.

COLLECTION

Collecting silybum is an experience! Find a good population of milk thistle, and bring cardboard boxes, five-gallon buckets, clippers, and most important, thick gloves. Cut the heads with less than 1 inch of stem and place them in buckets, transferring them to the boxes as needed. Look for heads that have finished flowering and are now showing a profusion of white pappus parachutes, for these contain the ripest seeds.

Seed samples from wild California silybum plants in different developmental stages were sent to Dr. Liersch, Dr. Vogel's colleague from Dr. Madaus and Company. His analysis showed the more mature heads contained seeds that had a substantially higher silymarin content. According to Liersch, the Silybum seed vessel, or *pericarpium,* is the only part of the plant to contain the silymarin (4–6 percent).

If one waits too long after the heads have opened, some of the seeds will be taken by the wind from the middle of the heads, leaving only the seeds around the edge. As many as one-half of the total seeds are lost when the head is past the optimum point. The peripheral seeds seem to be an adaptive feature of the plant. They remain in the heads late into the winter, when they fall and reseed the population. The windborne seeds will spread the plants to other areas.

Many species of birds are attracted to the seeds for food. In the summer it is common to see them clinging to the spiny stalks and swaying in the wind as they eat.

RECIPES

The seeds can be ground in a coffee grinder and eaten by the tea-spoonful—the most delicious and healthful way to add silybum to the diet. I often pull seeds right from wild heads wherever I find them and chew them up; they are delicious and provide a good taste treat and energy boost.

The kernel itself contains starch, protein, and fixed oil. The oil is up to 60 percent linoleic acid, an essential fatty acid (EFA) needed for prostaglandin synthesis. Recent studies have shown that adding foods rich in linoleic acid to the diet in high enough concentration can reduce chronic inflammation in the body by increasing the synthesis of prostaglandin PGE1. Other benefits of EFAs include helping to regulate female hormonal balance and reducing the possibility of cardiovascular disease, which is still the number one cause of death in this country.

Here are a few other ideas for adding this healthful plant to the diet:

All parts of the plant are edible, especially the young tender leaves and the stalks, which can be eaten raw or cooked. Only the spiny margins of the leaves need to be trimmed away, as they do not grow elsewhere. Silybum has a rich tasty flavor and is quite nutritious. The heads can be eaten cooked like those of its relative, the artichoke, although artichokes should be used with more caution. Finally, the roots may be baked or steamed and taste somewhat like salsify. Other ways to use the seeds:

- Soak the seeds overnight in water and puree in an electric blender. Strain off the starch "milk" and store in quart jars in the refrigerator. This can be drunk by itself or used as a substitute for other liquids in baking recipes. It is high in starch and oil.

- Take the drained, ground seeds, roast them in the oven, and add salt or herbs to make silybum gamasio—a seasoning salt.
- Brew the ground seeds with roasted dandelion or chicory to make a delicious hot drink to benefit the liver.

MEDICINAL PREPARATIONS

To maximize the concentration and accessibility of silymarin for medicinal use, make a tincture with the dry, powdered seed. Silymarin is soluble in ethyl alcohol and nearly insoluble in water, so a high percentage of ethyl alcohol to water should be used for the menstruum: 95 percent if available. Ninety-five percent alcohol is sold in some states under the name "Clear Spring." The tincture should be bright yellow, which indicates the presence of a resinous fraction containing silymarin. The name *flavonoid* comes from *flavus,* meaning "yellow."

SPECIFIC USES

Specific indications for the tincture are for any liver-based problem: cirrhosis, jaundice, hepatitis, weakened liver from drug or alcohol abuse, or liver poisoning from other foreign chemicals. Congested spleen or lymph can also be benefited, according to the Eclectics. Use it to strengthen the liver, in conjunction with other liver herbs, such as *Cynara scolymus* (artichoke leaves), *Taraxacum officinale* (dandelion root and leaves), *Artemisia vulgaris* (mugwort), *A. californica* (coast sage), and *A. capillaris* (the Chinese herb capillaris). *Bupleuriim* or *Scutellaria* (scute), other Chinese herbs, are also valuable.

After several years of using milk thistle extract, I have been able to improve my digestion and liver function, which was less than optimum after having hepatitis twice, 20 years ago. I take extra, up to 1 dropperful of the tincture or 1 tablet of the powdered concentrate three times a day, when my digestion is feeling weak—for instance, if I experience mild diarrhea or constipation due to overeating, wrong food combinations, eating while tired, and so on. This remedy has greatly benefited me and usually brings quick relief if I combine it with a regimen of light eating (mostly fruits and vegetables) for 5 days or a week. Light, circular, clockwise massage of the bowel and liver area is also helpful.

I have also heard some good stories concerning the benefits of milk thistle from health professionals around the country. In one case, a woman of forty was experiencing pain in the liver area as well as other symptoms of liver imbalance, such as poor appetite and headaches. She went to a medical doctor, who, after a series of tests, diagnosed chronic active hepatitis. He mentioned that she should see her banker, a blunt reference to the fact that this was a serious disease. It is worthwhile to note that liver disease is the fourth most common cause of death in this country.

Soon after this diagnosis, the woman heard about milk thistle and began taking it daily, 3 or 4 tablets (of the concentrated extract) as well as making some important dietary changes (see Dietary Recommendations below). Several weeks later she went back for more liver tests and the doctor was astonished to find that the enzyme levels (enzyme tests are one indication of the state of functional balance of the liver) had dropped to nearly normal! His only comment was that "there must have been a mistake in the first tests." Two months later I met this woman and she told me that she had been feeling better than she had for some time. This story is not an isolated incidence I am happy to say.

One medical doctor I have been in contact with has used milk thistle extract in his daily practice for three years. He has had good success (up to a 50 percent cure rate) with psoriasis, a disfiguring and uncomfortable skin ailment. He feels that this disease is liver and bowel related.

Although these experiences are anecdotal, they are about people who have been treated by trained health professionals using modern diagnostic tests. In Europe, milk thistle is commonly prescribed by medical doctors for many liver-related imbalances and is a favored medication. It is interesting that from 40 to 50 percent of all medical doctors in Germany use phytotherapy in their daily practice.

It seems certain that milk thistle and other well-documented herbal remedies, such as hawthorn and valerian, will soon take an important place in this country's medicine chest.

Dosage

The standard dose of 80 percentage standardized milk thistle extract is 60–120 mg, twice daily with meals. If you have hepatitis or need a stronger dose for added protection, I recommend up to 240 mg, twice daily, or even up to 360 mg, three times daily, for up to a week or ten days at a time, if you have a special need. In my herbal clinic, I have supervised many patients taking up to about a gram a day (in 2 or 3 doses) and have seen few, if any, side effects. Even this high dose was well tolerated. Occasionally patients reported a slight loosening of stools with higher doses, which completely resolved once the dose went back to a more usual 120 mg twice daily, which is a good maintenance dose. Studies show that silymarin is poorly absorbed from the intestinal tract and that the body eliminates it quickly, up to one-half in as little as 4 hours. That's why it's better to take milk thistle three times daily, with breakfast, lunch, and dinner.

Some milk thistle products contain a silybin-phosphatidylcholine complex. Some studies show that the silybin (1 part of the silymarin complex) is better absorbed when phosphatidylcholine is present, but these products often cost more. I always recommend that patients compare the cost, because if a straight silymarin product is half of the cost of one that contains phosphatidylcholine, the latter is not a good value. Just take 30 percent more of the silymarin product to make up for the less efficient absorption. If the prices were similar, however, I would try the complex.

DIETARY RECOMMENDATIONS FOR LIVER AILMENTS

When the liver is under any kind of stress, and especially during specific liver disease, such as cirrhosis or hepatitis, it is important to watch the diet closely. Too much oil and fat, especially when processed or cooked, is hard on the liver. The best oil is olive oil—avoid margarine and animal fat.

Red meat is also hard on the liver, as are drugs of any sort, alcohol, and cigarette smoking. Avoid processed foods in general, and focus instead on whole, fresh vegetables (lightly steamed), whole grains, and slightly sprouted, cooked legumes (such as aduki beans). At least one serving of vital green leafy vegetables a day, such as collards, Swiss chard, or beet greens, is highly desirable.

It is fortunate that milk thistle has moved to this country and is becoming so abundant and widespread. With drug and alcohol abuse on the rise, and with the number of synthetic chemicals in our environment increasing, our livers are under more stress. As the numbers of milk thistle increase, we may be counting our blessings instead of cursing them.

Notes

PART ONE: HOW THE LIVER WORKS

Farnsworth, N. R. 1980. Botanical sources of fertility-regulating agents: chemistry and pharmacology. *Progress in Hormone Biochemistry and Pharmacology,* vol. 1. Lancaster, England: Eden Press.

Personal Communication, May 1987, National Clearing House on Drug Addiction. *U.S. Statistical Abstracts,* 1984.

Raloff, J. 1993. EcoCancers. *Science News* 143:10–13.

Salbe, A. D. and L. F. Bjeldanes. 1985. The effects of dietary Brussels sprouts and *Schizandra chinensis* on the xenobiotic-metabolizing enzymes of the rat small intestines. *Food Chem. Toxic* 23:57.

Sixth Special Report to the U.S. Congress on Alcohol and Health, Jan. 1987.

Ukomadu, C. 2001. Alcohol and hepatitis, part 1 (http://www.veritasmedicine.com).

PART TWO: NATURAL THERAPY FOR THE LIVER

American Medical Association. 1986. *Drug Evaluations.* Chicago: American Medical Association.

Anonymous. 1980. Free-radical damage in the liver. *Free Radicals in Biology,* vol. IV, 49.

Bragg, P. 1976. *The Miracle of Fasting.* Santa Barbara: Health Science.

Chang, H. M., et al. 1985. *Advances in Chinese Medicinal Materials Research.* Philadelphia: World Press.

Chang, H. M. 1986. *Pharmacology and Applications of Chinese Materia Medico.* Philadelphia: World Scientific.

Cheung, C. S. 1983. The liver and gall bladder. *J. Am. Col. Trad. Ch. Med.* 2:30.

Davis, B., et al. 1985. *Conceptual Human Physiology.* Columbus: Charles E. Merrill Publishing Co.

Hikino, H. 1986. Antihepatotoxic actions of *Allium sativum* bulbs. *Planta Medico* 163.

Hobbs, C. 1992. *Foundations of Health.* Capitola, CA: Botanica Press.

Rose, R. C., et al. 1986. Transport and Metabolism of Vitamins. *Federation Proceedings* 45:30.

Salunkhe, D. K., et al. (n.d.), Anticancer agents of plant origin. *CRC Critical Reviews in Plant Sciences* 1(3):218.

Tiantong, B., et al. 1980. A comparison of the pharmacologic actions of 7 constituents isolated from *Fructus schizandrae. Chinese Med. J.* 95, A1–47.

Veith, I. 1972. *The Yellow Emperor's Classic of Internal Medicine.* Berkeley: University of California Press.

Vogel, A. 1926. *The Liver.* Bioforce-Verlag Teufen, Switzerland.

PART THREE: PROGRAMS FOR SPECIFIC COMPLAINTS

Bensky, D., and A. Gamble. 1986. *Chinese Herbal Medicine, Materia Medico.* Seattle: Eastland Press.

Bensky, D., and R. Barolet. 1990. *Chinese Herbal Medicine—Formulas and Strategies.* Seattle: Eastland Press.

Bradley, P. R. 1992. *British Herbal Compendium,* vol. 1. Dorset, England: British Herbal Medical Association.

Felter, H. W., and J. U. Lloyd. 1898. *King's American Dispensatory.* Cincinnati: The Ohio Valley Co.

Fratkin, J. 1986. *Chinese Herbal Patent Formulas—A Practical Guide.* Santa Fe: Shya Publications.

Hsu, H.-Y., et al. 1986. *Oriental Materia Medico, A Concise Guide.* Long Beach, CA: Oriental Healing Arts Institute.

Kaptchuk, T. J. 1983. *The Web That Has No Weaver.* New York: Congdon & Weed.

Kimura, Y., et al. 1984. Studies on *Scutellariae Radix,* IX—new component-inhibiting lipid peroxidation in rat liver. *Planta Medica* 50:290.

Kimura, Y., et al. 1985. Effects of extracts of leaves of Artemisia species and caffeic acid and chlorogenic acid on lipid metabolic injury in rats fed peroxidized oil. *Chem. Pharm. Bull.* 33:2028–34.

Kiso, Y., et al. 1985. Mechanism of antihepatotoxic activity of Wuweisisu C. and Gomisin A. *Planta Medica* 331–34.

Leung, A. Y. 1980. *Encyclopedia of Natural Ingredients.* New York: John Wiley & Sons.

Maeda, S., et al. 1985. Effects of Gomisin A on liver functions in hepatotoxic chemicals-treated rats. *Japan J. Pharmacol.* 38:347–53.

Maiwald, L. 1987. Bitterstoffe. *Zeitschrift fur Phytotheropie* 8:186–88.

Reynolds, E. S. 1980. Liver and biliary tree. *Systemic Reactions to Injury by Environmental Agents* 248.

Tierra, M. 1988. *Planetary Herbology.* Santa Fe: Lotus Press.

Yeung, H.-C. 1985. *Handbook of Chinese Herbs and Formulas,* 2 vols. Los Angeles: Institute of Chinese Medicine.

PART FOUR: HEPATITIS, CIRRHOSIS, AND FIBROSIS

Chuah, S. Y. 1996. Liver biopsy—past, present, and future. *Singapore Med. J.* 37:86–90.

Churchill, D. R., et al. 1996. Fatal hemorrhage following liver biopsy in patients with HP/infection. *Genitourinary Med.* 72:62–64.

Esteban, R. 1993. Epidemiology of hepatitis C virus infection. *J. Hepatol.* 17:S67–S71.

Gordon, S. C., et al. 1992. Lack of evidence for the heterosexual transmission of hepatitis C. *Am. J. Gastroenterol.* 87:1849–51.

Lindor et al. 1996. The role of ultrasonography and automatic-needle biopsy in outpatient percutaneous liver biopsy. *J. Hepatol.* 23:1079–83.

Little et al. 1996. Image-guided percutaneous hepatic biopsy: effect of *Ascites* on the complication rate. *J. Radiol.* 199:79–83.

Merck and Co., Inc., Caturelli, E., et al. 1996. Percutaneous biopsy in diffuse liver disease: increasing diagnostic yield and decreasing complication rate by routine ultrasound assessment of puncture site. *Am. J. Gastroenterol.* 91:1318–21.

Murphey, F. B., et al. 1988. Ct- or sonography-guided biopsy of the liver in the presence of *Ascites:* frequency of complications. *Am. J. Roentgenol.* 151:485–86.

Ohnishi, K., et al. 1996. Interferon therapy for chronic hepatitis C in habitual drinkers in comparison with chronic hepatitis C in infrequent drinkers. *Am. J. Gastroenterol.* 91:1374–79.

Okazaki, T., et al. 1994. Efficacy of interferon therapy in patients with chronic hepatitis C: comparison between nondrinkers and drinkers. *Scand. J. Gastroenterol.* 29:1039–43.

Oshita, M., et al. 1994. Increased serum hepatitis RNA virus RNA levels among alcoholic patients with chronic hepatitis. *C. Hepatol.* 20:1115–20.

Osmond, D. H., et al. 1993. Risk factors for hepatitis C virus seropositivity in heterosexual couples. *JAMA* 269:361–65.

Soyer, P., et al. 1993. Ultrasound-guided biopsy in focal lesions of the liver. Report on an automated biopsy system. *J. Radiol.* 74:215–19.

Stone, M. A., and J. F. Mayberry. 1996. An audit of ultrasound-guided liver biopsies: A need for evidence-based practice. *Hepatogastroenterol.* 43:432–43.

Thomas, D. L. 1995. Sexual transmission of hepatitis C virus among patients attending sexually transmitted diseases clinics in Baltimore: an analysis of 309 sex partnerships. *J. Infectious Diseases* 171:768–75.

Tobkes, A., and H. J. Nord. Liver biopsy: review of methodology and complications. *Digestive Disorders* 13:267–74.

Ukomadu, C. 2001b. Hepatitis C, Current treatments: overview.

Weinstock, H. S. et al. 1996. Hepatitis C virus infection among patients attending a clinic for sexually transmitted diseases. *JAMA,* 269:392–94.

Zhao, X. P., et al. 1995. Infectivity and risk factors of hepatitis C virus transmission through sexual contact. *J. Tongfi Med. Univ.* 15:147–50.

APPENDIX: MILK THISTLE

Abrams, Leroy, and Ferris, Roxana. 1960. *Illustrated flora of the Pacific States.* Palo Alto, CA: Stanford University Press.

Allain, H., et al. 1999. Aminotransferase levels and silymarin in de novo tacrine-treated patients with Alzheimer's disease. *Dement Geriatr Cogn Disord.* 10(3):181–5.

Angulo, P., et al. 2000. Silymarin in the treatment of patients with primary biliary cirrhosis with a suboptimal response to ursodeoxycholic acid. *Hepatology* 32(5):897–900.

Aurora, D. 1980. *Mushrooms Demystified.* Berkeley: Ten Speed Press.

Bunout, D., et al. 1992. Controlled study of the effect of silymarin on alcoholic liver disease. *Rev Med Chil.* 120(12):1370–5. Spanish.

Buzzelli, G., et al. 1993. A pilot study on the liver protective effect of silybin-phosphatidylcholine complex (IdB1016) in chronic active hepatitis. *Int J Clin Pharmacol Ther Toxicol.* 31(9):456–60.

Chan, M. K., et al. 1989. Hepatitis B infection and renal transplantation: The absence of anti-delta antibodies and the possible beneficial effect of silymarin during acute episodes of hepatic dysfunction. *Nephrol. Dial. Transplant.* 4:297–301.

Committee on Scholarly Communication with the People's Republic of China. 1975. *Herbal Pharmacology in the Peoples Republic of China.* Washington, D.C.: National Academy of Sciences.

Culpepper, N. 1847. *The Complete Herbal.* London: Thomas Kelly.

Deak, G., et al. 1990. Immunomodulatory effects of silymarin treatment in chronic alcoholic liver disease. *Orvosi Hetilap* 24:1291.

Ellingwood, F. 1983 (1898). *American Materia Medica, Therapeutics and Pharmacognosy.* Portland, OR: Eclectic Medical Publications.

Gerard, J. 1597. *Gerard's Herbal.* London: John Norton.

Grieve, M. 1981 (1931). *A Modern Herbal.* New York: Dover Publications.

Gunther, R. T. 1968 (1655). *The Greek Herbal of Dioscorides.* New York: Hafner Publishing Co.

Kunkel, Steven L., et al. 1978. Suppression of chronic inflammation by evening primrose oil. *Prog. Lipid Res.* 20:885–88.

Lang, I., et al. 1990. Immunomodulatory and hepatoprotective effects of in vivo treatment with free radical scavengers. *Ital J Gastroenterol* 1990 Oct;22(5):283–7.

Merck and Co., Inc. *The Merck Index,* 9th ed. Rahway, N.J.: Merck and Co. (Silybin).

Müzes, G., et al. 1990. Effects of silymarin (Legalon) treatment on the antioxidant defense system and lipid peroxidation in patients with chronic alcoholic liver disease: A double blind study. *Orvosi Hetilap.* 131:86. Neumaier, W. 1970. *Arztl. Praxis.* 21:3637.

Pares, A., et al. 1998. Effects of silymarin in alcoholic patients with cirrhosis of the liver: results of a controlled, double-blind, randomized and multicenter trial. *J Hepatol* 28(4):615–21.

Personal communication with the Poison Control Center, San Francisco, CA (phone call, August 1984).

Sonnenbichler, J., et al. Influence of silybin on the synthesis of macromolecules in liver cells. In *Proceedings of the International Bioflavonoid Symposium,* Munich, FRG:1981, p. 477.

Strubelt, O. 1980. The influence of silybin on the hepatotoxic and hypoglycemic effects of praseodymium and other lanthanides. *Arzneim.-Forsch.* 30:1690–94.

Szilagyi, I., et al. 1982. Isolation and structure of silymonin and si-landrin, two new flavanolignans from *Silybum marianum* (L.) Gaertn., Flore Albo. *Stud. Org. Chem.* (Amsterdam) 11:345–51.

The Bible. Genesis 3:18.

Velussi, M., et al. 1997. Long-term (12 months) treatment with an anti-oxidant drug (silymarin) is effective on hyperinsuline-mia, exogenous insulin need and malondialdehyde levels in cirrhotic diabetic patients, *J Hepatol.* 1997 Apr;26(4):871–9.

Voemel, A., et al. 1977. The lipid and flavonoid contents in the seeds of *Silybum marianum* Gaertn. under extremely varied eco-logical conditions. *Z. Acker-Pflanzenbau* 144:90–102.

Vogel, G. 1977. Natural substances with effects on the liver. In *New Natural Products and Plant Drugs with Pharmacological, Biological or Therapeutical Activity.* New York: Springer-Verlag, pp. 251–65.

Vogel, G. 1981. A peculiarity among the flavonoids—silymarin, a compound active on the liver. In *Proceedings of the International Bioflavonoid Symposium,* Munich, FRG:1981

INDEX